THE CONSENT GUIDEBOOK

A Practical Approach to Consensual,
Respectful, and Enthusiastic Interactions

Erin Tillman

authorHOUSE®

AuthorHouse™
1663 Liberty Drive
Bloomington, IN 47403
www.authorhouse.com
Phone: 1 (800) 839-8640

Published by AuthorHouse 02/28/2018

ISBN: 978-1-5462-3096-0 (sc)
ISBN: 978-1-5462-3095-3 (e)

Library of Congress Control Number: 2018902481

Print information available on the last page.

This book is printed on acid-free paper.

Dedicated to all Survivors.

CONTENTS

As an Inclusive Dating Empowerment Coach, NLP Practitioner, Author, and Speaker for over 10 years, I have coached singles in the realm of boundary-setting, self-improvement, and finding like-minded individuals who have similar relationship goals. Throughout my career, it has become more and more apparent that consent and boundaries can be tricky in the early months of dating when individuals are starting the process of getting to know each other. The more that I explored the topic of consent, it became clear that boundaries were not only being crossed in the dating scene, but also between colleagues, friends, and even family members.

We are currently interacting with each other partially based on our unique upbringings and past relationships. We can no longer assume that everyone has learned certain rules around what is considered to be 'appropriate' or 'inappropriate' behavior. Because there are few structures in place where the majority of individuals can learn the basics when it comes to consent and boundaries, it is of paramount importance that we start learning, teaching, and sharing fundamental ideas to encourage respectful behavior.

The conversation around consent is currently in a massive state of evolution. With the fierce momentum of the #MeToo movement throughout 2017, it has become clear that the conversation around consent is in the process of a major evolution and is being brought to the forefront of social awareness. In some cases, there is confusion as to what is and what isn't sexual harassment. For the first time in modern history, society as a whole has expressed outrage at what has been uncovered in regard to boundary-crossing, sexual harassment, and sexual assault.

We are entering an era where society is collectively saying that it's no longer ok to turn a blind eye when it comes to boundary-pushing and boundary-crossing and we are collectively calling for change. Within this emerging environment, people are becoming less and less afraid of speaking up about violations. Because consent has not been a topic that our society has had an open and honest discussion about in the past, we are currently finding our footing with these issues.

More insightful questions are being asked around consent and how to interpret verbal and non-verbal cues in a variety of social interactions. While consent and boundaries may be discussed differently in various communities and subcultures, it's clear that there is a vital need for more consent-based education overall. I believe that, generally speaking, there is a learning curve when it comes to consent and boundaries, meaning that respecting boundaries can also be learned and taught. At this moment, new societal norms are being created in regard to interacting with each other, establishing our own boundaries, and respecting the boundaries of others.

This Movement is bigger than any one expert. To offer a variety of perspectives, I invited Sex Educators, Health Professionals, HR Managers, Civil Rights Leaders, and Thought-Leaders to contribute consent advice, stories, and 'aha' moments to this book to offer a variety of perspectives. You will see their advice sprinkled throughout this book.

The intention of this book is to contribute to current productive conversations around consent and to provide a practical, easy-to-follow framework that encourages improved education in regards to establishing boundaries and respecting the boundaries of others. It takes all of us

CHAPTER 1

What Is Consent?

- ASSOCIATED DEFINITIONS
- BOUNDARY BASICS

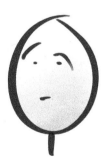

"*Waiting to teach about consent to young adults is too late. Consent-related behaviors should begin when children begin to talk and communicate their needs. Children who are raised in an environment that demonstrates, teaches, encourages, reinforces, and expects respectful social/human interaction is key. Allowing children to beg until they get what they want may seem like the norm in many families, but as you may imagine, it can set them up to believe that it's normal to beg for what they want until the other person gives in. It boils down to allowing them to coerce a person. Coercion is never okay. When seeking to fulfill a desire or need it's imperative that children are taught to ask first. May I....? Will you....? Would you like to....? Do you mind if....? These questions should be regular parts of their repertoire as they are growing up. Respectfully accepting the response they receive is equally important. Let's not forget that it is also important for parents to respect their child's level of comfort with social interaction and expressing affection. Shaming a child for not hugging or kissing a relative is contrary to what we should be teaching. If we expect them to respect the feelings and comfort level of others, we must do the same for them.*"

- Molly J Wray, Health Teacher

Boundary-pushing is not specific to age or gender. Anyone can be a boundary-pusher just as anyone can be a victim of boundary-pushing. Having said that, it is important to be aware of systemic hierarchies that exist in our society that can derail accountability. Whether intentional or not, your behavior may affect others and set an example for those around you. Your actions make an impact not only on your life, but also on the lives of others.

Your desire to feel safe is just as important as someone else's need to feel safe. It is reasonable to expect to be able to go through the day without having to defend oneself from other human beings verbally or physically. We all have the right to walk in this world not having to be harassed, touched, or groped by anyone without our permission.

Associated Definitions

There are many interpretations of the word 'consent'. Let's look at a few different definitions of the word 'consent' and other associated consent-based words that are used throughout this book. A few sources are included for some of the words where definitions differed.

Affirmative Consent- Explicit, informed, and voluntary agreement to participate in a sexual act. Both parties must give affirmative consent before sex. (Oxford Dictionary)

Affirmative Consent- Affirmative consent (enthusiastic yes) is when both parties agree to sexual conduct, either through clear, verbal communication or nonverbal cues or gestures. It involves communication and the active participation of people involved. This is the approach endorsed by colleges and universities in the

U.S., who describe consent as an "affirmative, unambiguous, and conscious decision by each participant to engage in mutually agreed-upon sexual activity. By definition, affirmative consent cannot be given if a person is intoxicated, unconscious or asleep. (Wikipedia)

Cisgender- *A term relating to, or being a person whose gender identity corresponds with the sex the person had or was identified as having at birth. (Merriam-Webster Dictionary)*

Cisgender- *Cisgender (often abbreviated to simply cis) is a term for people whose gender identity matches the sex that they were assigned at birth. Cisgender may also be defined as those who have a gender identity or perform a gender role society considers appropriate for one's sex. (Wikipedia)*

Consent- *Permission for something to happen or agreement to do something. No change may be made without the consent of all the partners. (Oxford Dictionary)*

Consent- *Getting permission for touching, kissing, or various sexual behaviors; Consent culture is becoming a wider-spread movement especially within feminist settings. If one does not have consent for a said act, the act is often considered sexual assault. (Urban Dictionary)*

Consent- *In common speech, consent occurs when one person voluntarily agrees to the proposal or desires of another. (Wikipedia)*

Entitlement- *Belief that one is deserving of or entitled to certain privileges. (Merriam-Webster Dictionary)*

Entitlement-*The belief that one is inherently deserving of privileges or special treatment. (Oxford Dictionary)*

Informed Consent- *Permission granted in full knowledge of the possible consequences, typically that which is given by a patient to a doctor for treatment with knowledge of the possible risks and benefits. (Oxford Dictionary)*

Informed Consent- *Informed consent can be said to have been given based upon a clear appreciation and understanding of the facts, implications, and consequences of an action. Adequate informed consent is rooted in respecting a person's dignity. To give informed consent, the individual concerned must have adequate reasoning faculties and be in possession of all relevant facts. Impairments to reasoning and judgment that may prevent informed consent include basic intellectual or emotional immaturity, high levels of stress such as post-traumatic stress disorder (PTSD) or a severe intellectual disability, severe mental disorder, intoxication, severe sleep deprivation, Alzheimer's disease, or being in a coma. (Wikipedia)*

Intentional Community- *A planned residential community designed from the start to have a high degree of social cohesion and teamwork. The members of an intentional community typically hold a common social, political, religious, or spiritual vision and often follow an alternative lifestyle. They typically share responsibilities and resources. Intentional communities include collective households, co-housing communities, co-living, ecovillages, monasteries, communes, survivalist retreats, kibbutzim, ashrams, and housing cooperatives. New members of an intentional community are generally selected by the community's existing membership, rather than by real-estate agents or land-owners (if the land is not owned collectively by the community). (Wikipedia)*

The #MeToo Movement- *"Me Too" (or "#MeToo", with local alternatives in other languages) spread virally in October 2017 as a hashtag used on social media to help demonstrate the widespread prevalence of sexual assault and harassment, especially in the workplace. It followed soon after the public revelations of sexual misconduct allegations against Harvey Weinstein. The phrase, long used by social activist Tarana Burke to help survivors realize they are not alone, was popularized by actress Alyssa Milano when she encouraged women to tweet it to "give people a sense of the magnitude of the problem". Since then, the phrase has been posted online millions of times, often with an accompanying personal story of sexual harassment or assault. The response on Twitter included high-profile posts from several celebrities, and many stories of sexual violence were shared. (Wikipedia)*

Restorative Justice- *An approach to justice that personalizes the crime by having the victims and the offenders mediate a restitution agreement to the satisfaction of each, as well as involving the community. This contrasts to other approaches such as retribution, deterrence, rehabilitation, or incapacitation. Victims take an active role in the process. Meanwhile, offenders take meaningful responsibility for their actions, seizing the opportunity to right their wrongs and redeem themselves, in their own eyes and in the eyes of the community. In addition, the restorative justice approach aims to help the offender to avoid future offenses. The approach is based on a theory of justice that considers crime and wrongdoing to be an offense against an individual or community, rather than the State. Restorative justice that fosters dialogue between victim and offender has shown the highest rates of victim satisfaction and offender accountability. (Wikipedia)*

Sex-Positivity- *Sex-positivity is an attitude towards human sexuality that regards all consensual sexual activities as* *fundamentally healthy and pleasurable, encouraging sexual pleasure and experimentation. The sex-positive movement advocates these attitudes. The sex-positive movement also advocates sex education and safer sex as part of its campaign. Part of its original use was in an effort to get rid of the frightening connotation that the term 'positive' had during the height of the AIDS epidemic. The movement generally makes no moral distinctions among types of sexual activities, regarding these choices as matters of personal preference. (Wikipedia)*

Sexual Assault- *Sexual assault is an act in which a person sexually touches another person without that person's consent, or coerces or physically forces a person to engage in a sexual act against their will. It is a form of sexual violence, which includes rape (forced vaginal, anal or oral penetration, or drug-facilitated sexual assault), groping, child sexual abuse, or the torture of the person in a sexual manner. (Wikipedia)*

Sexual Assault- *The action or an act of forcing an unconsenting person to engage in sexual activity; a rape; (Law) a crime involving forced sexual contact, variously defined as inclusive or exclusive of rape. (Oxford Dictionary)*

Sexual Harassment- *Sexual harassment is bullying or coercion of a sexual nature, or the unwelcome or inappropriate promise of rewards in exchange for sexual favors. In most modern legal contexts, sexual harassment is illegal. As defined by the United States Equal Employment Opportunity Commission (EEOC), "It is unlawful to harass a person (an applicant or employee) because of that person's sex." Harassment can include sexual harassment or unwelcome sexual advances, requests for sexual favors, and other verbal or physical harassment of a sexual nature. (Wikipedia)*

Sexual Harassment- *Behavior characterized by the making of unwelcome and inappropriate sexual remarks or physical advances in a workplace or other professional or social situation. (Oxford Dictionary)*

Sexually Transmitted Disease- *Any of various diseases or infections that can be transmitted by direct sexual contact including some (as syphilis, gonorrhea, chlamydia, and genital herpes) chiefly spread by sexual means and others (as hepatitis B and AIDS) often contracted by nonsexual means — called also STD. (Merriam-Webster Dictionary)*

Sexually Transmitted Infection- *Sexually transmitted infections (STI), also referred to as sexually transmitted diseases (STD) and venereal diseases (VD), are infections that are commonly spread by sexual activity, especially vaginal intercourse, anal sex and oral sex. (Wikipedia)*

Stealthing- *The practice of one sex partner covertly removing a condom, when consent has only been given by the other sex partner for condom-protected safer sex. (Wikipedia)*

"We start learning about consent as children. 'Is it OK if I give you a hug?' 'Do you still want to be tickled?' Silence, or laughter, is not an enthusiastic yes!"

- Lydia M Bowers, Sex Educator
LydiaMBowers.com

Boundary Basics

For those of you who might still be trying to engage in and understand this conversation about consent and boundaries, it boils down to this basic level of respect: My body is not yours to touch without my permission, and your body is not mine to touch without your permission. At the fundamental level, it goes back to what we hopefully learned as kids…do not touch or take what isn't yours. If it's not your property, whether that property is a tangible item or your body, you don't have permission to touch it or take it. If there's ever confusion, go back to that rule. "Do I have permission to touch that person's body?" If the answer is NO or even 'I don't know,' then don't go there, period.

Everyone's boundaries are different, which is why self-awareness is so important when interacting with each other. Maybe you know someone who might like it when you kiss them on the cheek to say hello. Consider that not everyone is going to feel comfortable with that. Even if you think this interaction is 'not a big deal,' to someone else, a kiss hello and being in close proximity could be very scary and possibly even cross a cultural boundary. It's about being adaptable and considering the other person's feelings. If you'd like to get to know someone better, practice asking for permission and waiting for their response, before proceeding with them.

As a general rule of thumb, you should not touch anyone who does not express an enthusiastic YES to being touched by you. It doesn't matter 'what you think they want' in regards to your interactions with them. Rather than assuming that someone is ok with you touching them, first get their consent to touch them or don't touch them at all. Your desire to touch someone should NEVER be more important than someone's level of comfort in regards to their own body being touched. You do not own any other individual's body and therefore it is not your place to touch them without permission. By putting yourself in the other person's shoes and stepping back from your own desires, you will better understand that not everyone's boundaries and feelings are the same as yours. In a consensual interaction, you are actively caring about how your actions are making someone feel.

Bottom line: Don't force anyone to interact with you, watch you, touch you, or be touched by you. Being overly aggressive or persistent in trying to get someone to say YES is not being respectful to their NO or MAYBE. Using someone's gender, sexual orientation, career, or lifestyle to push or make assumptions about someone's boundaries is not ok! We all deserve respect.

CHAPTER 2

Consent In Everyday Life

- DEALING WITH BOUNDARY PUSHERS
- BOUNDARIES WITH FAMILY
- BOUNDARIES WITH FRIENDS
- BOUNDARIES WITH COLLEAGUES

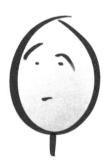

"Enthusiastic, continued consent needs to be present in kink, sex and platonic interactions. Take 'the hugger' for example. You've met them, they generally come careening toward you, saying, 'Oh, I'm a hugger!' and before you know it, they have wrapped their arms around you, pressed their body against yours . . . and squeezed. UGH!

It initially seems like a foreign concept; to ask, to check in, to state what you want, but weirdly, this typically leads to more enjoyable encounters in all realms of your life."

- Justine Cross, Professional Dominatrix
LosAngelesDominatrix.com

Verbal and non-verbal communication is the basis for all interactions with friends, family, and colleagues, not just romantic encounters. Hugs, hand-holding, a kiss on the hand, or even a kiss on the cheek can involve getting permission, too. When expressing interest in engaging with someone, asking *May I/Can I* questions AND paying attention to their verbal and non-verbal answers is important when determining someone's level of interest or engagement in an activity with you. Let's talk about hugging, for example. For some individuals, a hug from a stranger might not be a pleasant experience. Don't assume everyone wants to be touched or hugged. Don't force a hug. Get verbal consent for a hug when approaching someone by asking, "Could I give you a hug?" Wait for an answer before you proceed with a hug. A great way to initiate a hug non-verbally is to hold your arms out for a hug and let them meet you halfway, so they are able to make that decision of whether or not to engage in a hug with you. This protects you and the person you'd like to share a hug with...the hugger and the huggee. Same with a handshake! Offer your hand and let that person meet your hand halfway if they'd like to shake it. It's very important to not assume that everyone wants a physical interaction, even if we think that it's 'not a big deal.' It's always important to ask.

Everyone's boundaries are different, which is why it's important to not make assumptions when interacting with new people or even people you know. What if someone had a broken arm you didn't know about and you just grabbed them and hugged them without asking? You'd probably feel terrible that you might have hurt them by hugging them before they had the chance to tell you that they had a physical injury. It shouldn't take a physical injury for us to have empathy and to proceed with caution in regards to someone's physical comfort and/

or boundaries. It's their body; therefore, they should have the ultimate say as to how others interact with them physically, just as you should be able to feel comfortable expressing your boundaries if you are not interested or not able to engage with someone physically.

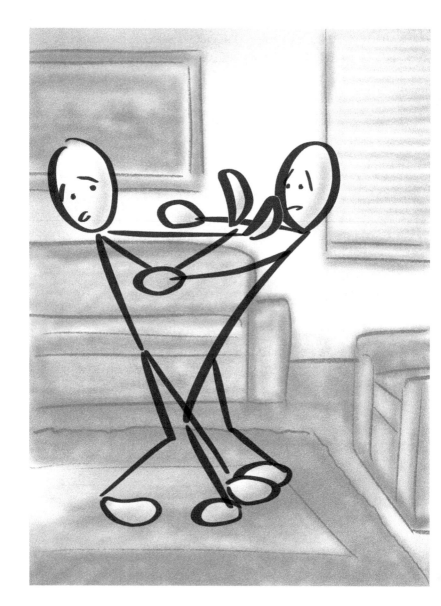

Dealing With Boundary-Pushers

For too long, we have been teaching each other to 'be polite' and not 'cause a scene' when people push our boundaries. It's important that we unlearn 'politeness' when it comes to protecting ourselves. We need to stop putting the possibility of 'hurting other people's feelings' above our own comfort and safety. If someone is being aggressive toward you, they should be aware of it, and you have the right to protect yourself against pushy, aggressive, or violent behavior.

Boundaries With Family

For many reasons, it can be difficult to set boundaries with family members. You can set boundaries with pushy family members by applying the 'safety in numbers' rule. Ask another family member to keep an eye out for you and have your back at family events if your uncle decides to interrogate you about your life choices, or your aunt starts questioning your political beliefs. A family member who is privy to potential boundary-crossing can interject and calm a situation or even whisk you away if you feel trapped. If you are feeling outspoken, respectfully telling a boundary-crossing family member about your new boundaries is a direct way to make your boundaries known. Be prepared that your family might feel entitled to tell you how they feel about your new boundaries or even tell you that they don't like these new parameters. Just remember that no one deserves to be subjected to triggering behaviors like being forced to engage in one-way conversations, having to defend oneself while not choosing to be an active participant in a debate, or being touched in any way just to make someone else happy...even friends and family members.

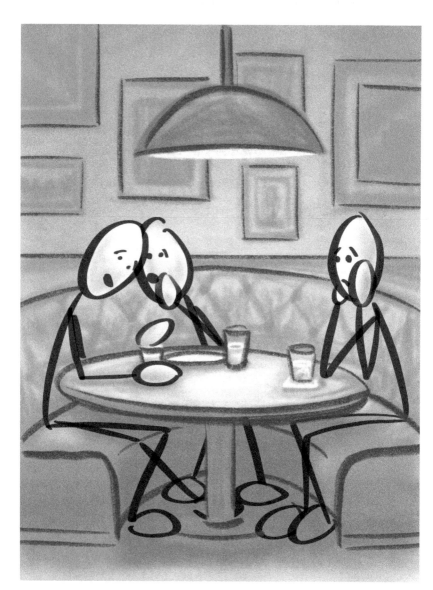

Boundaries With Friends

Sometimes people take liberties because you are friends. Just because someone is a friend doesn't mean that you should give up your levels of comfort for the sake of the friendship. Yes, friendship is caring and sharing, but not if that caring and sharing infringes on you or your friend's boundaries. True friendship shouldn't mean that one person sacrifices their own boundaries to make the other person happy. If a friend consistently acts selfishly and your comfort, safety, and physical or emotional boundaries are not being taken into consideration, it might be time to set new boundaries and in some cases, reassess that friendship. A friend who doesn't respect your boundaries isn't a true friend. A real friend will respect you and your request to shift your boundaries without making you feel bad for taking care of yourself. You should have each other's best interests at heart.

Boundaries With Colleagues

Establishing boundaries with colleagues can be complex. Though it's generally frowned upon to get too familiar with colleagues in a work environment, it's common to become friendly with those we interact with on a daily basis. Some companies have policies against hierarchal dating in the workplace to avoid a negative power dynamic where a person might feel pressured to accept a date, or be afraid to decline a date for fear that they could be punished or penalized for not going along with something a colleague is suggesting. It can be difficult to confront a colleague about boundary-crossing behaviors if you had a cordial, or even friendly interaction with them before an incident occurred. This becomes exponentially more difficult if it could possibly interfere with your career, livelihood, and potential for advancement.

If a colleague is overstepping your physical boundaries, there are a few things you can do to set new ones. Try suggesting that you'd prefer engaging in a different kind of interaction. For example, if you would prefer a handshake to a hug, a good strategy could be to reach out your hand first to demonstrate that you'd prefer to shake hands. Do what you can to remove yourself as much as possible from interacting with the colleague if they are not respecting your boundaries. Maybe it's possible to ask another colleague or manager for assistance, or asking if a shift or team assignment could be arranged. This could help avoid a confrontation with a colleague who might not understand why you are setting new boundaries. Your boundaries are your business, but sometimes individuals can feel offended if someone is questioning their behavior. Having said that, if you don't feel comfortable confronting a colleague on your own, it might be necessary to involve a third party. This could involve confiding in a trusted colleague or even reporting an incident to Human Resources. Ultimately, it's important for you to feel as safe as possible in your workplace.

CHAPTER 3

Digital Consent

- **RESPECTING BOUNDARIES WITH PHOTOS & VIDEOS**
- **COSPLAY & CONSENT**

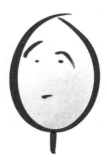

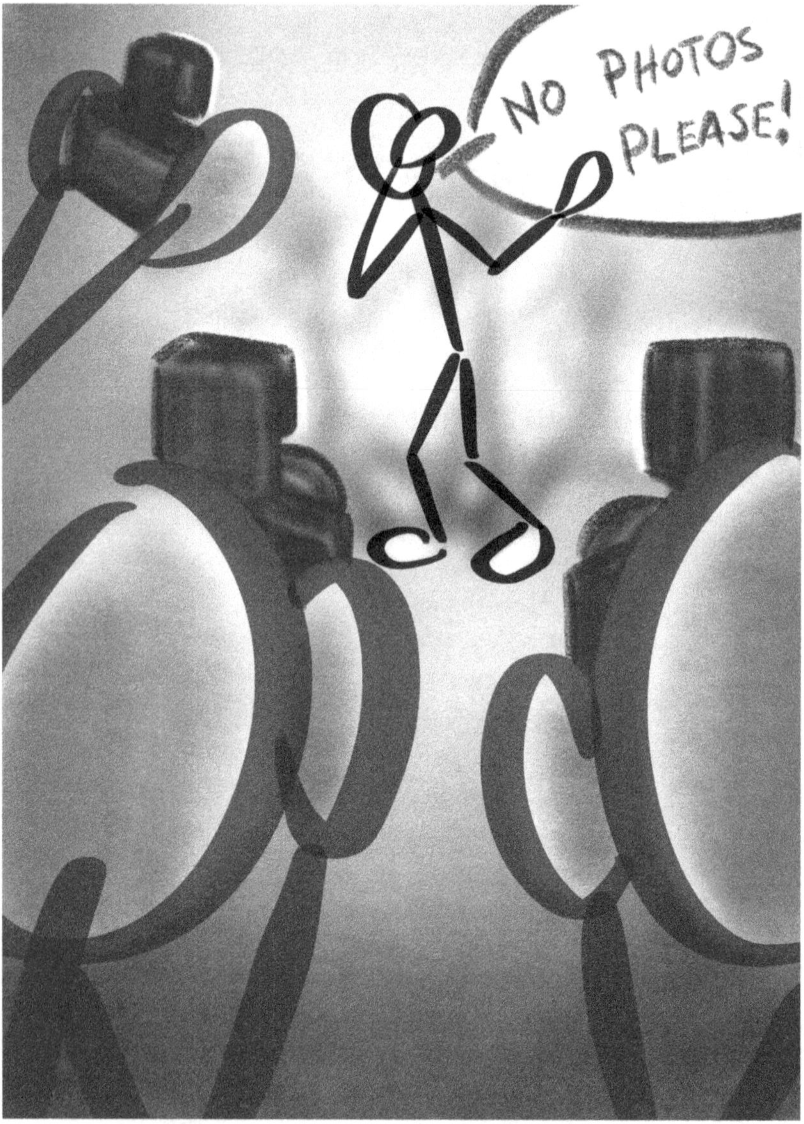
NO PHOTOS PLEASE!

Respecting Boundaries With Photos & Videos

We live in a selfie-driven society, but even so, not everyone wants their photo taken. Even if your intention isn't to post the photo or video to a public forum, some people might not want their photo taken, depending on the nature of the environment, and especially in a party scenario. Some individuals might have a job where, if certain photos are circulated, it could have a negative effect on their career or it could even cause unnecessary drama or conflict with their family, friends, or loved ones. Either way, it's not up to you to decide what someone should or shouldn't be ok with. That is up to each individual, and you should always have their consent before taking and/or distributing images.

1) *No posting or tagging individuals in photos or videos on social media without their consent!*

We are in an era where a lot of people will take photos of people for the intention of posting them publicly on various websites or apps. It's important that you get permission BEFORE taking a photo of someone AND before sharing it. You might think a specific photo is harmless, but the person in the photo might not want to be publicly associated with the other individuals in the photo, what is going on in the photo, or the site where the photo is posted. To be safe, assume that people don't want a photo of themselves floating around or posted somewhere without their permission. This also goes for posting group photos on dating app or dating sites. If you are going to post group photos on a dating site or app, be sure to ask your friend's permission to post those photos, and/or blur out their faces to respect their privacy while the world is swiping through your dating profile.

2) *Ask permission to take photos and videos of individuals at an event or party!*

If you are hosting a party or event, make an announcement so that attendees are aware that they could be photographed. If you'd like to go a step further and make your guests feel even more comfortable, you could give them the option of opting out of photos and videos altogether. This will allow your attendees to make a decision regarding participating or not participating in associated photos and videos taken at the event. Even better, ask individuals to sign a waiver saying that they are ok with being photographed while at the event.

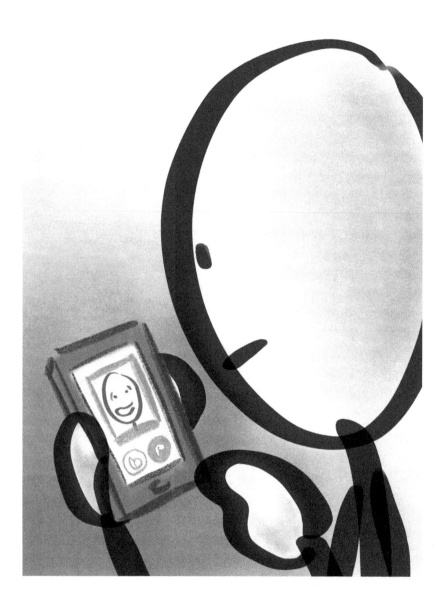

3) *No 'sexting' without consent!*

This should be a no-brainer, but, in case it's not, this is your gentle reminder that sending someone an unsolicited photo of your genitalia can be extremely upsetting to the recipient. Sexting and sending unwanted sexual photos is especially typical when meeting people on online dating sites and apps. No one should be forced to look at parts of your body, especially someone that you've just met, and ESPECIALLY if you haven't met each other yet. Also, if you do consensually choose to send sexy messages to someone, keep in mind that once those images are forever in the digital universe, you might not be able to control where they end up…. So be cautious about what photos and videos you are sending and who you are sending them to.

"As an actor and filmmaker, knowing that a set I'll be working on will be a safe environment is important to me and everyone involved. Whether it's stage combat or a steamy love scene, communication and consent are essential and should also be mirrored in real life."

- Jason Marsden, Actor/Filmmaker

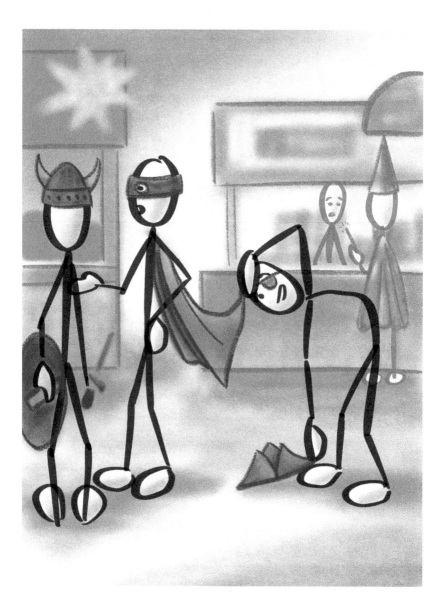

Cosplay & Consent

Costumed conventions can be a fun time, a place to escape reality and celebrate your favorite fictional characters. Imagine being in the realm of fantasy when, all of the sudden, you are touched inappropriately while celebrating comic books and your favorite super heroes with your friends. Even if someone is 'just' taking a photo with someone because their costume or character is awesome, it's important to get permission to take their photo or touch them in any way. Even if the goal of the photo is to pose with them in a way that feels like 'what their character would do,' it's important to remember that this is a real person in real life...NOT a character! A cool photo should not be more important than respecting someone else's boundaries. Just because it's a fun atmosphere, it doesn't mean that boundaries shouldn't be respected.

Because of the increased number of complaints, more and more comic & cosplay conventions have put measures in place to emphasize the importance of respecting boundaries, like creating their own Anti-Harassment Policies for their events and training the event staff to appropriately handle any incidents. New York Comic Con (NewYorkComicCon.com) has enforced a zero-tolerance policy for harassment and encourages attendees to "be respectful, be nice, be cool and be kind to each other." Their policy prohibits behavior including, but not limited to, physical assault and/or battery, harassing or non-consensual photography or recording, inappropriate physical contact, unwelcome physical attention, costumes that include hate symbols, and offensive verbal comments in general, but also associated with race, gender identity/gender presentation, sexual orientation, age, body size, or disability. This is their way of keeping these events fun, respectful, and safe for all attendees.

CHAPTER 4

The New Consent Standard

- WHY 'NO MEANS NO' IS PROBLEMATIC
- INFORMED CONSENT
- ENTHUSIASTIC CONSENT
- AFFIRMATIVE CONSENT & CALIFORNIA'S 'YES MEANS YES' LAW
- INTERPRETING NON-VERBAL CUES
- DEALING WITH HEARING NO (OR NOT HEARING YES)
- THE ASSUMPTION OF CONSENT & THE POP CULTURE CONNECTION

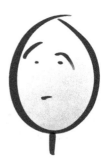

"We are currently reframing what consent means. 'NO Means NO' is the mantra for life! However, it should be reframed 'YES means YES!' Educating about consent on an enthusiastic level can and will be life-changing for many people in sex and in other activities in everyday life. 'MEH doesn't mean YES!' I am incredibly receptive and grateful to anyone who respects when I say NO the FIRST time."

- Nicole Holmes, Sexual Health Educator
Facebook.com/NickyHeartsPublicHealth

Erin Tillman

Why 'No Means No' Is Problematic

We grew up hearing 'No Means No,' and that it's our job to 'Say No' to stop someone else's actions against us. But why is the focus and responsibility put on the person whose boundaries are potentially being breached? Why aren't we doing a better job teaching individuals to be aware of their actions and showing people how to not be aggressive or pushy toward others? Not everyone has the capability to verbally say NO. Consider that some people might feel 'frozen in fear' and might not have the power to speak up and say NO. Others might not have learned to feel comfortable saying NO forcefully. Some people might not have the ability to communicate verbally in the way that you do. If, when getting to know someone, they express a specific way that they feel most comfortable conveying YES and NO, you can use that knowledge going forward when interacting with them. You can establish another mutually agreed upon way of communicating with them. Getting to know an individual's unique way of communicating can be easier when there is an established relationship, friendship, or prior interaction with that person. It's time to teach individuals how to be better at exercising self-control when it comes to boundary-pushing, rather than putting all of the weight on the more vulnerable person to take action, when it's their boundaries that are being crossed.

"Consent knows no gender. While it's clear men need to do a lot of work around consent, women and non-binary people can be culpable as well. We all need to improve our ability to recognize power differentials and practice using our words when it comes to sexual touch."

- Allison Moon, Author, Girl Sex 101
GirlSex101.com

"Consent is not only the acknowledgment of permission, but the understanding of boundaries around consent before engaging."

- Theresa Braddy, Therapist
Twitter @TheresaBraddy

"If you don't feel safe saying NO, then your YES becomes messy. You might feel violated, even after expressly giving verbal permission. Those feelings are valid and each person is responsible for the impact of their actions. Safe is a relative term, as nothing is free of risk and no encounter is 100% safe. Just as there is the phrase 'safer sex,' consent ranges from safer to riskier on a spectrum. Unlike physical barriers, the language of consent has no scientific percentages to measure effectiveness. The best we can do is reduce the risk of accidentally violating each other with empathy, reassurance, and actively reducing pressure associated with consent."

- Wry, Non-Monogamy Consultant
Polytalks.com

Informed Consent

In dating, informed consent is when communication is at its best and all parties involved agree to participate in a certain interaction. Informed consent is a meeting of the minds between individuals as to which specific interactions they are agreeing to. In a perfect world, all parties involved would also know exactly what each other's boundaries are and what exact actions and interactions they are potentially engaging in. Knowing the specifics of each other's boundaries can be tricky, especially in new relationships while you are still in the process of learning about each other's likes and dislikes. The more conversations you have, the more likely you are to avoid missteps than if you 'just go for it' and hope for the best.

Saying YES verbally can be helpful for those who are comfortable and able to use verbal communication to express their boundaries. It's important to be aware that some people aren't physically able, haven't learned, or are possibly just learning and getting comfortable with confidently expressing a verbal and/or non-verbal NO for various reasons.

"Remember the enthusiastic part of enthusiastic consent. This is paramount when giving or receiving consent. While every YES does not have to come with its own parade, it does have to come from a place of interest, excitement, and joyful curiosity. If one partner feels indifferent about the sexual experience, or agrees to go along out of a sense of guilt or obligation, that person is not giving their full consent. Enthusiastic consent requires actively making a choice rather than resigning yourself to one."

- Leigh Montavon, Sex Coach
Instagram @SexCoachLeigh

Instead of asking people for what they'll allow, ask people what they want. It is so important to the development of enthusiastic consent to agree on desires and not just consequences. Instead of, 'Is this ok?' or 'Can I?' consider asking, 'Would you like...?' Also, ask BEFORE touching someone, not AFTER."

- Irina Sarnetskaya, Filmmaker/Educator
IrinaSarnetskaya.com

"If someone does not give you an enthusiastic YES, ASK AGAIN! Silence is not a YES. 'MAYBE,' is not a YES. 'HELL YES,' is a YES. 'I would love to,' is a YES. And if you sense hesitation in their answer, ASK AGAIN! It does not hurt to make sure you are on the same page. ALWAYS!"

- Jimanekia Eborn, Sex Educator/Trauma Specialist
SEWJIM.com

"*The hottest first kiss I ever had happened on an 'accidental date' with a guy I'd known in my friend circle for about a year. We ended up volunteering together on the same overnight shift at a festival, and sat next to each other by a fire, talking and telling stories of our lives for a while. It was chilly, so we slowly moved closer together, and finally, after he finished a tale about his childhood dog, I looked him in the eyes and asked him, 'What would you do if I kissed you right now?' He smiled and said, 'I'd kiss you back.' And then we kissed. It was easily the hottest and most perfect first kiss of my life.*"

- Avens O'Brien, Libertarian Writer/Speaker/Activist
Avens.me

Enthusiastic Consent

After someone is informed and agrees to be a part of a specific interaction with you, they will hopefully be enthusiastic about your impending interaction. If someone is a MAYBE, it's unlikely that they are enthusiastic about the pending interaction. It's understandable if this is a new concept for many. In this new age of consent, it's important to engage with people who are enthusiastic to lessen confusion and potential misunderstandings associated with intimate encounters. It's likely that the more enthusiasm someone has, the more likely they are to be excited about future interactions with you. Besides, consensual and enthusiastic interactions are the most fulfilling. We should all be striving for enthusiastic interactions in all areas of our lives.

If someone is not an enthusiastic YES, it's a NO!

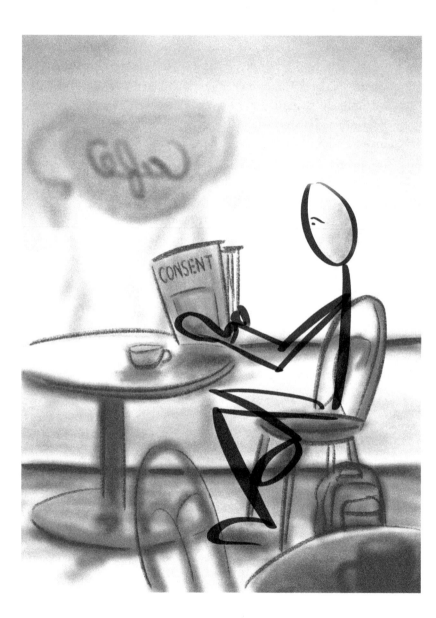

Affirmative Consent & California's 'Yes Means Yes' Law

California is the first state to create the *'YES Means YES'* law encouraging and enforcing affirmative consent. This law is designed to create a standard for consent and sex including *'empowerment programming for victim prevention, awareness raising campaigns, primary prevention, bystander intervention, and risk reduction'* on college campuses. This is a big step in a positive direction for consent-education.

The law approved by California Governor Jerry Brown in 2014 states that, *'Affirmative consent means affirmative, conscious, and voluntary agreement to engage in sexual activity. It is the responsibility of each person involved in the sexual activity to ensure that he or she has the affirmative consent of the other or others to engage in the sexual activity. Lack of protest or resistance does not mean consent, nor does silence mean consent. Affirmative consent must be ongoing throughout a sexual activity and can be revoked at any time. The existence of a dating relationship between the persons involved, or the fact of past sexual relations between them, should never by itself be assumed to be an indicator of consent.'*

*The entire bill can be viewed in it's entirety on the California Legislature Website at

https://leginfo.legislature.ca.gov/faces/billNavClient.xhtml?bill_id=201320140SB967

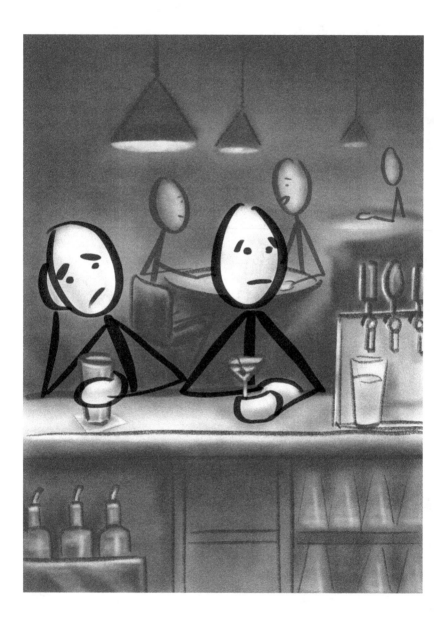

Interpreting Non-Verbal Cues

It's even more important not to push boundaries with individuals who are unable or uncomfortable expressing themselves verbally. If you are not sure that someone is an enthusiastic YES to a specific interaction (either verbally or non-verbally), it's best not to proceed. Each situation and interaction is different, but there are certain behaviors that can signal unease. Having said that, there are some non-verbal signals that someone might not be interested in engaging with you, (i.e., they are not an enthusiastic YES!).

1) Someone is backing away

If the person you are interested in engaging with keeps backing away while you are interacting with them, this might be a sign that they are not interested in continuing the interaction. At the very least, it might mean that they feel that you are too close in proximity to them.

2) *Someone is avoiding eye contact*

Lack of eye contact can sometimes mean shyness or nervousness, but it can also mean that a person could be disinterested in the interaction. At the very least, lack of eye contact does not indicate an enthusiastic interaction.

3) *Someone isn't responsive to verbal/non-verbal interaction*

A lack of responsiveness during a conversation can mean anything from confusion or lack of comprehension, to disinterest or annoyance. If someone isn't responding to your questions, isn't engaging in a back-and-forth conversation with you, and/or is 'frozen' in their interaction with you, it could be a sign that they are not interested in continuing a conversation with you at that moment in time.

4) *Someone seems distracted while interacting with you*

If someone is looking at other people, searching for others while talking to you, or seems generally distracted while talking to you, it might simply mean that this might not be a good time for this person to engage in a specific interaction with you. They might very well be interested in interacting with you later, if and when they are less distracted, but if they are not actively engaging with you at that moment, find others who are more present and enthusiastic about having a chat with you.

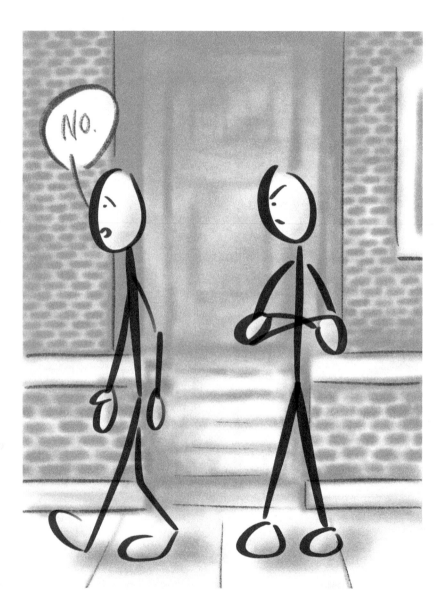

Dealing With Hearing NO (Or Not Hearing YES)

We need to unlearn entitlement where human interaction is concerned. We need to learn to be okay hearing, and gracefully accepting NO.

Be mindful of not directing feelings of anger at someone if they decline your offer to shake hands, hug, kiss, etc. Someone could have any number of reasons for not wanting to engage with you. Do not take it personally! There are infinite reasons as to why they might choose not to engage with you - anything from they are a germaphobe, to they are sensitive to touch, to they've had a prior traumatic experience and are selective about who they engage with in certain ways. You might not know why they seem uninterested in shared interaction with you and it honestly doesn't matter why. It only matters that their boundaries are respected. Consider that this person is doing you a favor by being honest about their level of comfort, or lack thereof, in that moment. Whether verbal or implied, their NO is a gift. If someone is not an enthusiastic YES, don't push boundaries. Everyone deserves to have an enthusiastic YES from everyone they are interacting with.

"Consent is necessary because it is hardwired in our experience of Self. Part of being is rooted in the possibility to make choices. The choices that we make allow us to express who we are, how we feel, and what we desire. Consent, then, flows out of our existence as interdependent, but autonomous, self-determined beings. A person's consent cannot be implied, it has to be actively and consciously chosen. Our participation in any experience is optional, and being given the space to exercise that choice is life-affirming. When denied the opportunity to freely give our consent, we inevitably feel less of our rightful humanity. We feel less valued, less seen, and most significantly, less safe. Any act that is void of consent is void of connection, and therefore also void of pleasure. So then it is also true that any experience that welcomes and holds space for enthusiastic, uncoerced, or even affectively neutral consent also holds space for authentic human connection and welcomes the possibility of pleasure."

- Shadeen Francis, Therapist/Educator/Author
ShadeenFrancis.com

The Assumption of Consent & The Pop Culture Connection

We make a lot of assumptions around consent, in part because of the human interactions we see in popular culture. Many things in films, TV, porn, and music do not translate to our real human interactions. We collectively have been basing our interpersonal interactions on fantasy...something that a writer or artist created to entertain us. Over and over again, we've seen romantic scenes in movies, where after many attempts, a hesitant woman 'gives in' to the sexual advances of the handsome, yet persistent, object of her affection. We consciously and unconsciously mimic these stories and attempt to use them in our own social interactions. We are led to believe that we can convince someone to make out with us. In some cases, we treat someone's personal boundaries as a game, challenge, or obstacle that is stopping us from getting to our own personal sexual goal. This kind of entitlement is learned behavior based on what we were taught growing up with pop culture. There's one major problem with this: We are real people with real boundaries, feelings, likes and dislikes, we are not characters in a TV show, movie, or song lyric. In reality, being sexually persistent when someone is hesitant is problematic on many levels, and is even considered to be a crime in certain cases. If our past interactions were based on what we learned from pop culture, gossip, and 'just going for it,' this new age of consent is based on communication, respect, and reality.

CHAPTER 5

Accountability

- TALKING WITH SOMEONE WHO HAS CROSSED BOUNDARIES
- HOLDING OTHERS ACCOUNTABLE
- GAINING AWARENESS THROUGH FEEDBACK
- POSSIBLE SOLUTIONS AFTER CROSSING SOMEONE'S BOUNDARIES

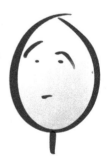

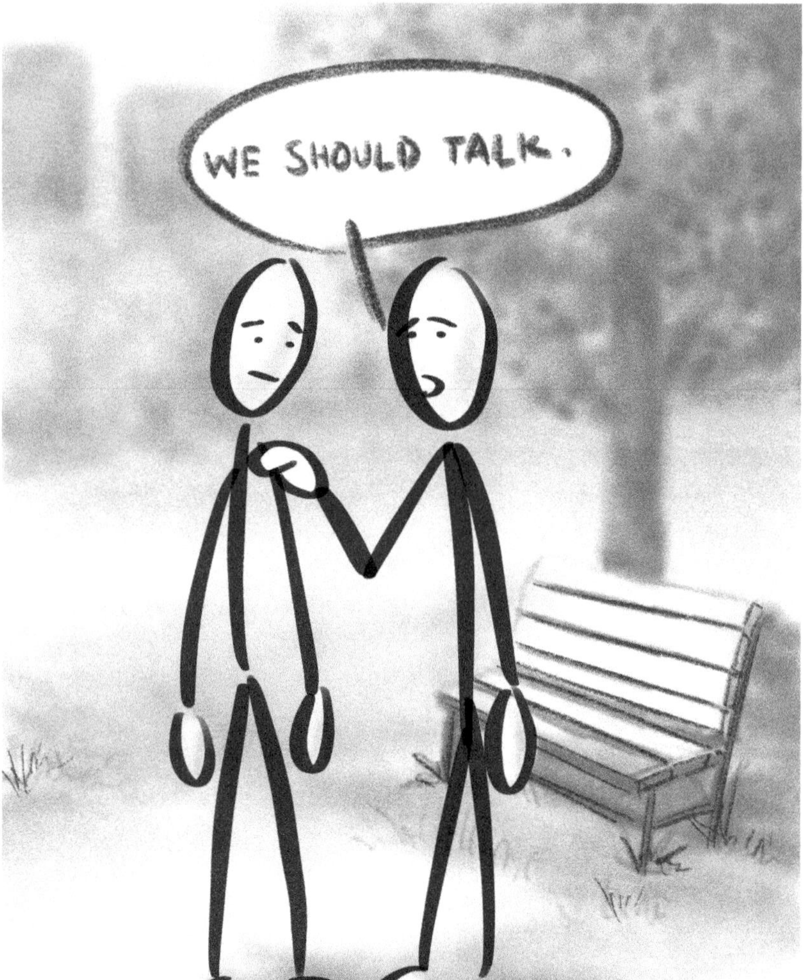
WE SHOULD TALK.

Talking With Someone Who Has Crossed Boundaries

What can you do if you hear or see someone pushing someone's boundaries? What if someone tells you that someone you know has violated their boundaries?

Silence enables the behavior. Whether you approach someone publicly or privately after you see, hear, or learn that an incident has occurred, it's important to speak up.

When expressing concerns about someone's words or actions, consider talking to them in a way in which they are more likely to listen to you. Your words can help the boundary-pusher see how their behavior negatively affected others.

So what can you do? Don't be an enabler! If you see something, say something to help stop the enabling and cycle of boundary-crossing, assault, and general disrespectful behavior toward others. Let's hold each other to a higher standard.

If you see that someone might be in distress and you feel like you can help out safely, there are a few things you could say to potentially help deescalate the situation. Here are a few specific examples of things you can say:

"Are you ok?"
"Is everything ok over here?"
"Can we talk for a second?"
"Do you need help?"

You could directly approach the person who feels uncomfortable directly and ask them, "Are you ok? Do you need help?" By addressing the 'victim,' you are letting all parties involved know that they are 'seen' and you are potentially someone who is looking out for them. Also, by addressing the 'victim,' the boundary-pusher will be made aware that someone is paying attention to what's happening. This can help to diffuse the situation in that moment. We don't know what will happen after the fact, but, in that moment, the victim knows that someone is there and paying attention to the interaction. A simple "Hey! Is everyone ok here?" can possibly help someone who feels trapped in an uncomfortable situation.

When approaching the boundary-pusher, it's important to do what you can to keep yourself as safe as possible. If the boundary-pusher becomes aggressive, combative or belligerent, it might be appropriate to ask others to help calm them down rather than go it alone. For example, if you are in a bar or club, alert the bartender or security. If you are at a friend's party, tell the host. Asking others to assist you in coming to someone's aid can help protect your safety as well.

Holding Others Accountable

If someone you know personally has pushed someone's boundaries, whether it's a friend, family member or a colleague, it is absolutely our obligation to speak up rather than be silent about their behavior. A great way to get their attention and help them to understand how their behavior might be potentially hurtful is to ask them how they would feel if the roles were reversed. Encouraging someone to stop and take a moment to picture themselves in the shoes of the person on the receiving end of their aggressive behavior, could be a helpful way to put things into perspective. Say something like: "Hey friend...That thing you said/did to that person in the bar was kinda weird. Let's talk about it. I'm your friend and I love you and I don't think that best represents who you are." If you show your concern by making it about them and wanting them to be better, they might be more apt to listen.

You might feel conflicted if you become aware that your friend or family member has crossed someone's boundaries. It is normal to feel conflicted. If you love them, the best thing you can do is to lovingly hold them accountable. Help them get help. If you want to support them, but you have conflicted feelings about their behavior, maybe the healthiest way for you to help them is to support them from afar. Enabling or ignoring their behavior will only add to the problem and potentially create a situation where others could be harmed.

None of this is easy. These conversations are uncomfortable for everyone. We need to become more comfortable with the discomfort. With practice, this will get easier. We owe it to ourselves. We owe it to our fellow brothers and sisters. We owe it to our community. We owe it to society. It's for the greater good. We're all in this together. Together, we can do better.

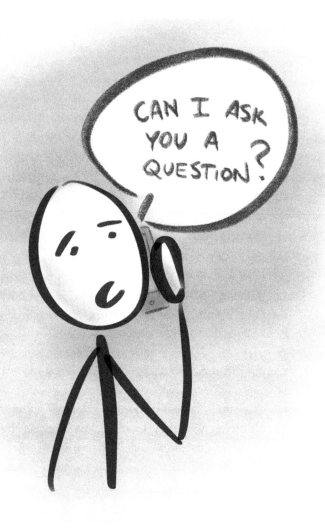

Gaining Awareness Through Feedback

Are you aware of your own behavior and how it affects others? One way to gain insight into our behavior is to ask those you've had close interactions with for feedback regarding your past interactions, positives and negatives in relation to how you interact with each other, and ways to improve interpersonal interactions so that everyone feels respected. Becoming aware of our own behavior and the impact that it has on others is a gift that can improve our future interactions. It may initially be hard to hear that our behavior has negatively affected someone, especially if that was not our intention, but once we've been made aware, we can make more intentional and respectful decisions in the future. We can all do better to be more intentional when it comes to relating and interacting with others. We have the power to change our behavior.

Possible Solutions After Crossing Someone's Boundaries

Other than going through the legal process, we currently don't have a ton of solutions in place when it comes to what happens after someone has been accused of sexual harassment or sexual assault. Here are some possible steps and solutions for someone accused of a boundary violation.

1. *Listen*

Listening is the first thing you can do when someone has made you aware that you have crossed their boundaries. You might have a variety of thoughts and feelings about what your accuser is saying about your actions, but before attempting to formulate an argument, rebuttal, or defense, listen to what they have to say. It will probably feel uncomfortable to hear that your actions could have caused harm, but avoiding, arguing, or denying the truth of what happened during a consent violation can do further harm. Do not brush off someone who you may have harmed. Listen to what they are saying and how they are feeling. At the very least, hearing how your actions are affecting others might be an opportunity for growth when interacting with others respectfully and harmoniously.

2. *Apologize And Ask What You Can Do To Start The Healing Process*

If you've crossed someone's boundaries, you may have to accept that they might not be able to accept your apology for one reason or another. Depending on the circumstances, the boundary-pushing may cause a great deal of pain and anguish to someone. This person may not be able to forgive you in the way that you would like, but everyone processes these situations differently. You may not get the reaction you were hoping for. Make it known that you are sorry and ask what you can do to make amends and start the healing process.

3. *Self-Awareness & Education*

What steps can you take moving forward to improve your interactions with others? Are there resources you can access to learn more about healthy and consensual interpersonal interactions? Answering these questions will take a willingness to honestly assess your behavior. If you can acknowledge that your actions might have caused harm, then you can start the process of gathering information to upgrade your interpersonal interactions and make more consensual decisions in the future.

4. Counseling/Therapy

There is no shame in asking for help. Seeking professional help can be an effective way to gain insight into current thought patterns and associated behaviors, and find ways to improve or change harmful behaviors. Gaining a new perspective and learning new tools from an objective party can be helpful for your growth in current and future interpersonal interactions.

5. Restorative Justice

If you are a part of an intentional community and an incident has occurred between you and another community member, restorative justice could be a possible solution, depending on the severity of the incident. This process involves the accuser, the accused person, and a third person (a community member) supportively holding space for, and participating in a conversation with the intention of creating understanding of the hurt caused and starting the healing process. This is only possible if all parties are willing to be active participants in the process.

CHAPTER 6

Consent Green Lights
& Red Flags

- 14 PRE-CONSENT QUESTIONS
- CONSENT GREEN LIGHTS & RED FLAGS
- EMOTIONAL INTELLIGENCE & CONSENT COMPREHENSION
- CONSENT UNDER THE INFLUENCE

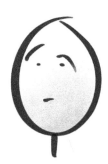

"In the game of life, we all want to play. Consent can be a fun social game where everyone can score. You wouldn't just toss a ball at someone; you would ask if they want to play Catch. So let's use CATCH as a way to check in and get consent.

C is for Chat or Compliment - Do they want to have a conversation or receive a compliment?
A is Associate - Do they want to be acquaintances, or more affiliated with you?
T is Touch - How, where, when, what are you asking to touch or be touched?
C is for Coitus - Are they interested in having sex & what does that look like?
H is for Hello, Head-nod, Handshake or Hug - How are we greeting others? Some people might not be ok with the standard social cue of extending a hand out as a greeting. So start with a Hello & find out what people are ok with.

It is my goal to see that CATCH catches on and makes for ease around social connections at the start so deeper consent communication happens more often, leading to the best game of life we can play."

- Christi Anne Bela, Intimacy Architect
Practical Happiness Living

14 Pre-Consent Questions

Feeling comfortable, safe, and respected by a new potential partner is super important and can eventually lead to you enthusiastically consenting to sexual activity. When getting to know a potential new partner, it can be stressful to initiate conversations about sex and intimacy. In a perfect world, we would all have a serious chat about boundaries before engaging in intimate acts. In fact, I highly encourage that. For those who might be shy about discussing specifics about sex, asking yourself a few questions before starting a consent/sexual boundaries conversation with a partner could help determine if a potential partner is a good fit for you. Here are 14 questions that can help you assess your possible level of comfort with a new potential partner. If your answer to any of these questions is negative, you may want to rethink your willingness to engage in sexual activity with someone new.

1. Do you feel physically safe with your potential partner?

2. Do you feel emotionally safe with your potential partner?

3. Does your partner respect your boundaries in normal scenarios?

4. Do you feel comfortable voicing your likes and dislikes to your potential partner?

5. Is your potential partner open to hearing your likes and dislikes?

6. Does your potential partner respect you when you say NO?

7. Does your potential partner respect your feelings overall?

8. Do you trust your potential partner?

9. Does your potential partner have good judgment?

10. Does your potential partner lose control when under the influence?

11. Is your potential partner concerned about your well-being?

12. Do you feel forced by your potential partner to try things you're not interested in?

13. Does your potential partner respect your friends and family?

14. Would you have any regrets after being intimate with your potential partner?

Avoid drama with a new potential partner by using these 14 questions to assess if a new potential partner is a good fit for you. If, after answering these questions, you still feel excited about the idea of getting it on with a new potential partner, you may be well on your way to consensual sexy times! Once you've chosen a partner that makes you feel comfortable and safe, the consenting part becomes way easier. Not to mention, safety and consent make every intimate encounter that much sexier. Before you make a move (or consent to letting your partner make a move), here are a few things to remember...

*Pay attention to your potential partner's behavior outside of the bedroom. Oftentimes a person's respect level is consistent regardless of the situation. For example, if someone isn't respecting you outside the bedroom, it's quite possible that they won't respect you while in the bedroom.

*If you are able, voice your concerns if something feels wrong to you at any time during both intimate moments and regular situations. Your partner is not a mind reader, so it's important to be clear about what your boundaries are or/and tell your partner if a personal boundary has been crossed, so that they can adjust their actions accordingly. Show and tell your partner what works for you so you can feel more comfortable in consensual intimate interactions. If your partner acts unsupportive or aggressive after you've expressed your concerns, boundaries and comfort level, do what you can to leave the situation safely.

*Tell a friend, roommate, or family member where you'll be and who you're on a date with just in case something unexpected happens. You don't want to be in a situation where no one knows where you are or who you're with.

"Civil Rights Activist Audre Lorde said, 'When we speak, we are afraid our words will not be heard or welcomed. But when we are silent, we are still afraid. So it is better to speak.' I believe Lorde's words are of vital relevance today as so many women are coming forward and using their voices to speak out against those who have violated their trust, their bodies, and their right to give or refuse consent. Women all over are standing up to say, "Enough!" Many we see televised and flooding social media and yet there are many more who stand using their voices without the spotlight cast upon them. These women stand boldly through hashtag campaigns such as #MeToo, or in their own corners of the world, to stand in solidarity while navigating their way through mountains and walls of fear to let their voices be heard. Men and women must clearly understand what it means to give and/or receive consent. It is also important that both understand that consent may change within one encounter. And just because consent was given previously does not indicate carte blanche. Consent includes paying close attention to body language and understanding the dissonance that may occur between what's being stated and body language. Now, more than ever, we all need to use our voices whether we fear that our words will be received or not. We need to begin initiating conversations by using whatever platforms we have available to us. NOW is the time to send the message that ALL women have the right to give or withhold consent without fearing the threat of retaliation and/or harm. Consent is RESPECT! Consent is Sexy!"

- Dr. Alicia M. Ellis, LPC-MHSP, Sex Therapist
Alicia Ellis Counseling & Consulting

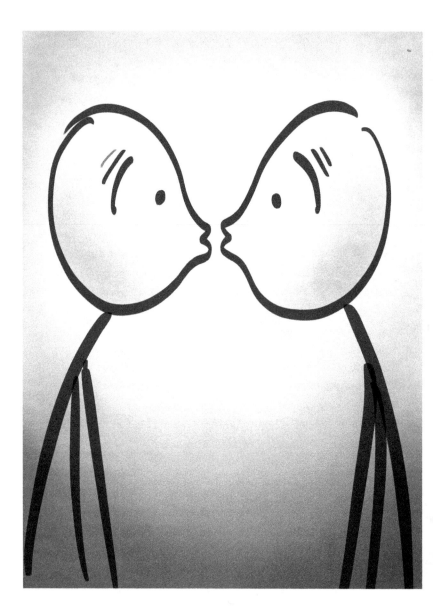

Consent Green Lights & Red Flags

It's often the little things that can make you feel the most respected with a new intimate partner. 'Green lights' are the opposite of 'red flags' in that they are positive signs that someone is committed to making your comfort a priority during intimate moments. Here are 7 things that can set the stage for consensual comfort with a potential intimate partner. Consider adding your own 'green lights' to this list that would make you feel more comfortable and at ease with a new intimate partner.

1. Respecting Someone's Venue Preferences

If a potential partner would feel more comfortable in a specific place, do what you can to make them feel as comfortable as possible. Being in a noisy environment, an apartment with distracting roommates, or even simply being in a new person's home can be stressful, especially for someone who already might feel nervous about the potential for an intimate encounter. Choosing a comfortable and inviting location can lessen anxiety and nervousness attached to venue distractions.

2. Respecting Someone's Body

Your partner's body is not a toy. There is a person attached to their body parts. It's important to stay present and conscious of the fact that the person you'd like to share intimate moments with has thoughts and feelings. You can do this by checking in with your partner throughout your intimate encounter to make sure you're both enjoying the experience.

3. Respecting Someone's Energy Level/Stamina

Shaming a potential partner for not having your level of energy, or what you consider to be an ideal amount of energy, is not ok. Accept the energy and stamina that they are able to bring to the experience.

4. Respecting Someone's Physical Capabilities Or Limitations

There may be some movements or positions that might be uncomfortable, or in some cases, not possible for an individual. Unexpectedly trying to maneuver your partner's body to do that acrobatic move you saw online is not consensual and could be quite painful. Respecting someone's physical abilities will make them feel more comfortable, and in turn, add to the level of comfort for everyone involved.

5. Respecting Someone's Preferred Form Of Protection/ Contraception

Contraception choices are highly personal for some people. Pressuring someone into not using their preferred method of protection, stealthing, or any other reversal of agreed-upon protection, is not consensual behavior. You could be potentially exposing each other to potential pregnancies or STI transmission. At the very least, you are going against the agreed upon method of protection which is potentially a breach of your intimate agreement. Just don't do it.

6. Respecting Someone's Sexual Pace

It's not a given that you and your partner will be interested in doing the same things at exactly the same moment. Stay present with them and check in regularly to make a mutual decision to keep things where they are or take things up a notch throughout an intimate encounter.

7. Respecting Someone's YES/NO/MAYBE List

If you have compared and discussed your YES/NO/MAYBE List with your partner (more on this in Chapter 7), then it's important that you respect each other's list. Yes, your lists might evolve or change, but it's important to respect what is currently in place. These lists can be fun, but they should also be taken seriously as an on-paper representation of your potential partner's boundaries, likes, and dislikes.

It is possible that you will have fewer options if choosing potential partners based on this list, but the remaining prospects will hopefully come with a higher level of respect and comprehension around boundaries, as well as an eagerness to make sure you feel comfortable in intimate scenarios. It's important to prioritize your comfort and safety in potential intimate encounters. Be wary of sacrificing your own comfort and safety to please someone else.

Emotional Intelligence & Consent Comprehension

We all have different levels of emotional intelligence and different levels of comprehension where boundaries are concerned. Consent is a very new concept for some. If you have a high level of consent comprehension, someone who is just learning about the idea of consent or might be having trouble understanding the importance of consent, might not be a good fit for you. It can be difficult to come to terms with the fact that a potential new partner, who we are excited about, might not be on the same page. It's important to acknowledge that some individuals might not be a good fit for you.

If you do see potential in someone and choose to invest time and energy to teach them or support them through the learning process, be kind and support them through as they learn new concepts and ideas. It's important that you be honest with yourself about how much time and energy you are willing to devote to their comprehension of personal boundaries, and specifically respecting your boundaries.

Be clear about what your emotional needs are and weed out people who aren't on your same emotional level. Choosing partners who have a similar level of emotional maturity can lessen misunderstandings. Your intuition can help guide you through the process of figuring out if you and a potential partner have different emotional needs.

Never disrespect someone because they aren't on the same level of comprehension. Their lack of understanding is not necessarily malicious. It just might mean that you have more knowledge and/or awareness around personal boundaries. There can be a learning curve regarding consent. If someone you would like to spend more time with is truly trying to understand, give them some time to process this shift in interpersonal interaction.

If while supporting your potential new partner in their journey to fully understand the concept of consent, you discover that fundamental differences still remain in the way you communicate, show respect, and process the idea of consent, it might be time to let them go as a potential intimate partner. If you do walk away, do so knowing that you gave this interaction a good try and even though the end result might not be what you had planned, you aided someone in their consent-educational journey.

"As a top, you should always pay attention to the reason your bottom is consenting. Do they just want to please you? Are they afraid to say no? Are they intoxicated? Or do they really want to consent."

- Mona Darling, Sex Educator/Kink Mentor
DarlingPropaganda.com

"I'm a cisgendered heterosexual male Social Justice Educator who champions the concept of consent. That said, I had WAY too much to drink one night at an open-bar party with co-workers. Frankly, I was drunk and don't remember the last half of the evening. I was informed a couple days later that I'd gotten 'handsy' with a couple different women. This was embarrassing and made me feel like a hypocrite for behaving differently than what I preach. For me, the only course of action was to apologize for my actions and to quit drinking altogether. This way I know I'll maintain control of my behavior at all times.

- Anonymous

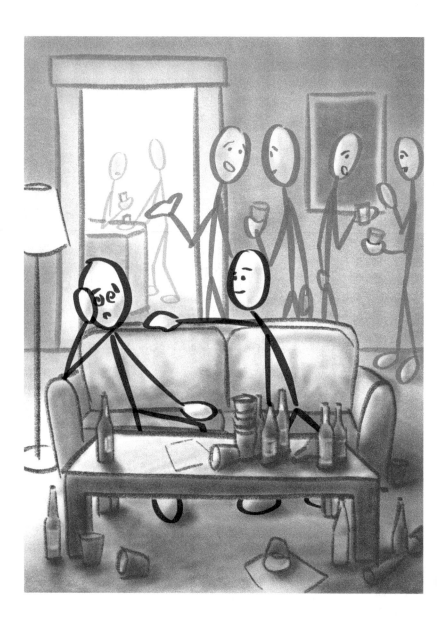

Consent Under The Influence

At what level of intoxication does consent become invalid? An individual's ability to give consent and assess someone's ability to give consent become blurrier when intoxicated. This goes for both the pursuer and the person being pursued. Because everyone reacts to alcohol and drugs differently, there is not one clear answer in regards to when someone is too intoxicated to give and assess someone's ability to give consent. Possible signs that someone is too intoxicated to give consent can include, but are not limited to, slurred speech, eyes that aren't focused, balance issues, staggering, alcoholic breath, and poor muscular coordination. There can be many other signs, but also someone could show none of these signs. Because there are no definitive behaviors that everyone exhibits, it's better to err on the side of caution and abstain from activities that involve giving consent, if it is unclear whether or not someone is fully able to give consent. Don't let your desire to pursue someone cloud your judgment, disregard someone else's boundaries and level of comfort, and put both of you in an unfortunate and potentially dangerous situation. Doubt means don't! It's not worth it!

CHAPTER 7

Sexy Consent

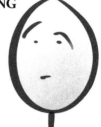

"Consent is UNCOMMON. I hadn't realized I actually needed it. I'd never given verbal consent and I'd also never received it. In May 2013, I found myself back on the dating scene after ending a six-year monogamous relationship. Although it was at my request, meeting at my place was sort of awkward for me. I was not comfortable at all. The guy I had been dating sat on the bed next to me, he gently tapped me on the shoulder and asked, 'Do you like to kiss?' I shook my head yes like those shy school girls you see in the movies. Then he continued, 'Would you like to kiss me?' It was the first time anyone had EVER asked me for access to MY BODY. After that, I was totally comfortable and the awkwardness dissipated. I've searched my memory in the years since trying to recollect another time when I was actually asked for my consent. I can't remember another time this has happened."

- Victoria Wray, Sexuality Blogger
PrettyPinkLotusBud.org

"Getting good at setting boundaries is a lot like training at the gym... It takes time and practice to build up our 'NO' muscles. It can help to practice with people you feel safe with, and make simple requests. A lot of people decide that because saying no is hard, they must be bad at setting boundaries. The truth is, most people haven't practiced saying no. It would be like going to the gym and deciding that because you can't lift 100 lbs, you're never going to be good at lifting weights. Give yourself and others the gift of a firm no. There is power in being able to trust that people will be honest with you about their boundaries and feel safe enough to share their truth with you. You can become the role model who inspires your family, community and workplace to be more authentic and have better boundaries."

- Cathy Vartuli, Emotional Freedom Coach
TheIntimacyDojo.com

"When we speak with the average Joe or Jane about consent, the number one question we hear is, 'Won't it be awkward to talk about this?' Our answer is usually, 'More awkward than getting naked and intimate with someone else's bodily fluids and genitals?'

Bottom line – sex IS awkward…and messy and beautiful. Talking about your wants and needs before getting down and delightfully dirty doesn't ruin any mood; rather it shows your potential partner that you respect yourself, respect them, and care enough to prepare for the experience of being intimate together.

As a bonus, talking with a potential partner may just open the door to experiences you didn't even know were open for discussion! When you charge in blindly, without a conversation, you have to guess what your partner wants and needs, and assume they are into it. When you talk about it all ahead of time you can focus, instead, on giving them exactly what they've asked for! We don't know about you, but both of us find it incredibly hot to know when we're pushing the right buttons. Consent is necessary and, though it doesn't have to be, verbal consent IS sexy even when it's awkward. Hearing 'Yes' come from your partner's mouth is sure to enhance the experience."

- Sean & Jennifer Rahner, Sex Educators
GeekySexyLove.com

"Something that I think can be helpful for discovering the wants, needs, and dislikes of a partner is discussing those things before engaging sexually. This conversation can be fun and flirty but also set up 'ground rules' for what sexual activities each person wants to participate in."

- Sarah Perry, Sex Educator
Facebook.com/SarahExplains

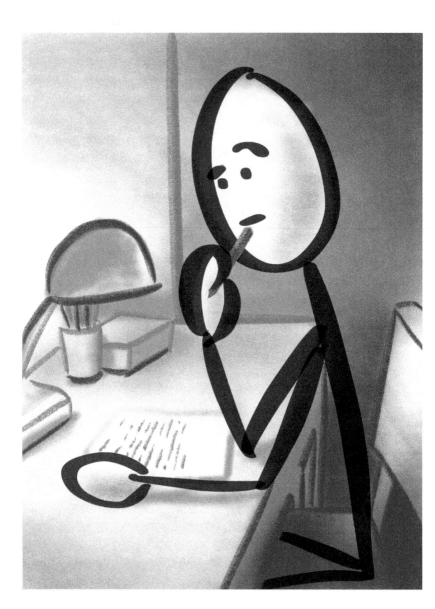

YES/NO/MAYBE: Empowerment In Boundary-Setting

There are a lot of ways you can get to know your boundaries and/or reassess your boundaries. For a lot of us, we upgrade our boundaries after they have been crossed. An upsetting incident can force us to revisit our boundaries in a dramatic way. Though incidents can happen even with clear boundaries in place, figuring out your boundaries in a variety of situations can be a good starting point when entering into new consensual interactions.

Several organizations have created helpful YES/NO/MAYBE lists to help you assess your likes and dislikes with things associated to sex and intimacy. These lists are a great starting point for figuring out your own boundaries, but can also be a fun way to start a conversation with a new partner, or revisit and refresh boundaries with an existing partner. Think of it as a sexual icebreaker. Teen Sex Ed online resource *Scarleteen* has a great YES/NO/MAYBE list on their website (**Scarleteen. com**). Although its core audience is 15-25 years old, it is a great resource for all ages when it comes to starting conversations about sex, sexuality, and intimate boundaries. Please be aware that a lot of the YES/NO/MAYBE lists online have content that is NSFW (Not Safe For Work), so use discretion when accessing these lists in public places.

There will be some things that are absolute NOs for you in all situations with all people. There will be some things that will be a NO for you in some situations, but a YES in other situations or with certain people. There may be some things that you might be a YES to with most people. It's up to you to decide what is on your YES/NO/MAYBE list. Again, the things on your list are allowed to shift and change. While you might be a YES to kissing your date goodnight tonight, you might be a NO to a goodnight kiss on another night. These lists can be a great starting point to get to know yourself and potential partners when appropriate, and when the time feels right to you.

A word of caution about the MAYBE category on YES/NO/MAYBE lists... Let's say that you are comparing lists with a potential partner and you see that your potential partner is a MAYBE to a specific interaction. A MAYBE means that your potential partner is currently undecided about engaging in this interaction, so it's important to treat that MAYBE as a NO for now, or until you have a follow-up conversation about it. Do not make assumptions about things on someone's MAYBE list. A MAYBE is not a consensual and enthusiastic YES.

"One beautiful thing about practicing consent is the power it gives to our yeses. If we aren't strong in our NOs, how can we stand firmly in what we DO want? Consent isn't only about boundary setting, but welcoming and embracing our desires while respecting the same for others."

- August McLaughlin, Author & Podcast Host
AugustMcLaughlin.com

"Consent is a muscle. We have to practice it to get better at it. Being a professional cuddler helps me practice it a lot; that makes it easier for me to ask for what I want, say YES and NO more freely, and get better at receiving both YESes and NOs. The more we get exposed to these conversations, the better our society will be at respecting our boundaries and asking for what we want."

- Yoni Alkan DHS, Sexual Educator
YoniAlkan.com

"Consider verbalizing the option of NO and let your partner know that you will still like them and want to hang out with them if they say NO. For example, 'I'd love to make out with you. I'm totally fine if you're a NO to that, or if you don't want to go there. And if you're a NO to that idea, I would still like to be friends.' This lets people know that you won't drop them if they give an answer they think you don't want to hear."

- Hunter Riley, Sex Educator
OutAboutSex.com

Practicing Saying NO

Saying NO isn't always easy depending on the scenario and the people involved. Practicing expressing NO in various scenarios can be helpful, but it's not a fail-safe. It's important to focus on teaching each other to respect boundaries and not be overly aggressive and/ or persistent with those we are interacting with. Hopefully we can all practice expressing our NO as well as respecting each other's boundaries. After all, practice makes perfect!

Once you start getting comfortable with your new established boundaries, the idea of speaking your truth and sharing your boundaries with others will get easier and easier. Knowing your own boundaries will make it easier to weed out those who don't respect them. Anyone who feels uncomfortable or offended by your boundaries is someone who does not deserve your time and energy.

If you are nervous, tentative, or having trouble expressing your boundaries verbally, here are a few ways you can practice feeling more empowered when it comes to verbal boundary setting:

1) Practice saying NO in front of a mirror. The first step in getting comfortable saying NO to others is to get comfortable saying the word NO in general. No can be a very difficult word for a lot of us, especially those of us who don't want to feel like we are 'disappointing' others. Getting more confident with your NO is you taking care of yourself, not you trying to please others by sacrificing your own levels of comfort.

2) Practice setting boundaries in all areas of your life, including when you meet new people in social environments, with colleagues, with friends, and with potential partners.

Start getting comfortable demonstrating your boundaries with new acquaintances. Practice saying NO to people and things that you're not an enthusiastic YES to.

3) Practice taking a moment to check in with yourself on a regular basis at various points in time, and during a variety of encounters to get in tune with what your true feelings are about a situation. This quick check in can happen at any time and in any situation. It could be right after a friend asks you for a favor. It could be the moment someone asks you out on a date. It could be in the middle of a sexual encounter. You are absolutely allowed to take a breath...pause...and proves how you really feel about a request, interaction, or encounter, before responding.

4) Give yourself permission to change your mind. It's ok to feel one way at the start of an interaction and feel another way later on during that same interaction. Feelings are not fixed. They are fluid and can change for an endless number of reasons. It is ok. It can be helpful to check in with yourself to tune into the fact that your feelings are changing and, if possible, *how* they are changing. Once you are aware of how you are feeling, it is then important to share those feelings with the person you are interacting with and/or remove yourself from the interaction to take care of yourself. Don't ignore your own feelings and boundaries for the sake of 'being nice' or not wanting to disappoint someone.

"Consent isn't just about asking for permission. It's about respecting the person in front of you enough to stop and contemplate their needs before your wants. The only way you'll truly know what those needs are is to have a conversation and, even then, you have to be open to respecting whatever answer you receive."

- Dirty Lola, Sex Educator/Host of Sex Ed A Go Go
SexEdAGoGo.com

"I had a dream where a man learned I was a professional cuddler and came over to get a hug. I said, 'Hold on a minute!' I wasn't ready for this hug. He paused briefly and then came at me again. 'Hold on,' I said! This was awkward. He tried two more times until he finally heard me and stopped. Later in the dream, we were hugging with consent. He cried because my saying no to him earlier was painful. I didn't feel guilty about it. I felt compassion for his experience. I knew his sadness could be a growth experience for him if he chose to see it that way. At Cuddle Sanctuary, we practice being gracious when a person says no to us. The phrase we suggest saying is, 'Thank you for taking care of yourself.' This phrase says so much. It says that sometimes the most important thing a person can do for themselves is set a boundary. Thanking someone for setting a boundary with me requires ninja-level maturity. It gets me out of my ego and reminds me that this other person in front of me has needs. And sometimes, those needs are distance. From me."

- Jean Franzblau, Consent & Sex-Positive Speaker
SexualEsteemWithJean.com

Respecting & Validating The Boundaries Of Others

When someone tells you their boundaries, respect them. It is not your place to shame anyone for their personal boundaries. Respecting your potential partner's boundaries is imperative to positive, productive, and mutually pleasurable encounters. Once blaming and shaming enters into the picture, the pleasure level decreases for one, if not both potential partners. Our society shames and blames people for their lifestyle choices, which is hard enough. The last thing your potential partner needs is more blaming and shaming from you, the person they are potentially going to be intimate with. Support your partner by accepting their personal boundaries and not making them feel bad about their personal limits. Being respectful of your potential partner's boundaries will greatly lessen the potential for harmful encounters and will make your partner feel respected, accepted, and supported. Supporting your partner's boundaries will set you up for successful consensual interactions.

Here are a few simple ways that you can support someone's boundaries:

1) SHARE your YES/NO/MAYBE lists. Acknowledge that you hear, understand, and support the person's boundaries by saying, "Thank you for taking care of yourself."

2) CHECK IN regularly with your partner during intimate interactions to make sure they are comfortable. Have an open dialogue. Most issues occur when assumptions and generalizations are made.

3) RECAP and have conversations after your interactions to see if your impressions of how things went match your partner's experiences.

4) ASK for feedback. Is there anything you can specifically do to better support each other's boundaries going forward?

The effort made here will show a partner that you are serious about wanting to make sure that they feel comfortable with you. That effort alone will make an individual feel more comfortable and might have the unintentional result of them wanting to spend more quality time with you in the future!

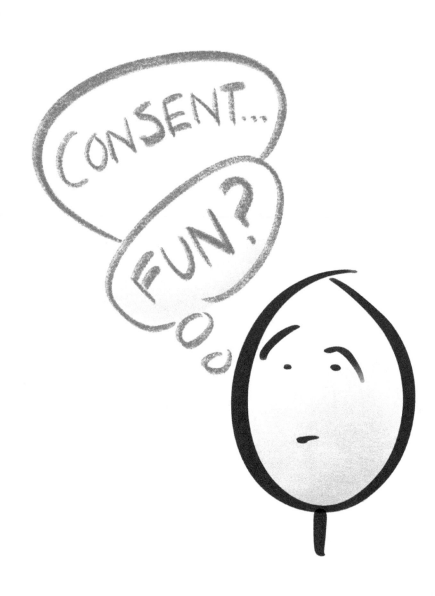

Making Consent Fun

Who says consent and related conversations have to be hard or scary? Consent conversations can be fun if you use them as a sexy way to get to know your potential partner. A flirty convo about your sexual likes and dislikes can help determine your intimate compatibility, plus this conversation can be a turn-on in and of itself. Have a conversation before engaging with someone to learn potential likes and dislikes. There are many sources online that involve YES/NO/MAYBE checklists that detail a variety of things that you each can go through in a fun way to figure out where the two of you have similarities and common interests. These discussions can be difficult, but YES/NO/MAYBE lists can make these conversations fun and casual. Keep in mind that even if your partner says that they are into what you are suggesting at that point in time, it doesn't necessarily mean that they will always be into it. Checking in with your partner prior to all encounters - especially romantic encounters - can be helpful in terms of knowing boundaries. Communicating with your partner before and/or during each sexual encounter is very important. Also, even if someone says that they are into something, they always reserve the right to change their mind at any point during the sexual encounter. Human beings are not one-dimensional. These conversations and interactions flow from one encounter to the next. Just like you might not want vanilla ice cream for dessert after every meal, someone you interact with might not want the same intimate interaction with you every time you are together. This is why it's so important to be present and have a check-in conversation to get clear on what you and your partner are into at that point in time.

"Consent is an underlying part of boundaries, which is crucial to all our relationships. Overstepping boundaries, including sexual boundaries, is a form of abuse. We tend to confuse or muddy the messaging about consent and abuse of all types. We should be teaching young women and men to set and enforce boundaries. That includes verbal and physical boundaries. But that does not, and should not, place the responsibility or 'blame' on anyone victimized or abused. I had to learn how to set boundaries as an adult, so I made sure to teach my own daughters from a young age about setting boundaries. I never insisted upon blind loyalty or that my children never question me 'because I am the parent.' From a social perspective, we expect girls to obey, to be 'good girls.' This makes it awfully difficult for women to set boundaries. Another issue that confuses consent is false-virgin status, when women pretend to be shocked that a guy would suggest sex, so that he can twist her arm or pour her another drink as though we're living in a Jane Austen novel. NO means NO, not, 'Well, pour me another shot of tequila and let's see how it goes.'

I am a professional writer and my 'turf' includes politics, health, and transition post-divorce, as well as embracing a confident single life. From a professional and personal position, the issues of consent, assault, harassment, and abuse are extremely important to me. I have seen women re-enter dating after long marriages or relationships with no idea how to set boundaries, sexually or otherwise. For some women, the lack of strong boundaries, combined with a former abuser who trampled over any attempts to set boundaries, led to divorce. I've advised women to use online dating to practice setting boundaries. If something doesn't feel right to you, say so. You've got nothing to lose. Most of the time, when we have difficulty setting boundaries, it's because we're afraid of rejection or that we won't be liked. Use online dating to figure out what's acceptable to you and what's not. There is no standard answer.

Dating & Sex: Listening, Observing, And Checking In

Another crucial element to giving and receiving respect is being able to listen. Listening to your partners before, during, and after intimate moments will help you to understand their level of comfort, likes, dislikes, and things that can be adjusted or improved in your interactions. To be an effective communicator is to be able to listen. Becoming an amazing intimate partner takes listening. Listening can involve noticing words and sounds your partner is making during an intimate encounter, but also watching your partner's body movements. Nothing is more irritating than someone who isn't listening to our needs, wants, and desires during sex and intimate moments. Conversely, it's a complete turn on to be with an intimate partner who is listening and interested in your pleasure as well as theirs. We might be so excited to have the opportunity to be with a partner that we forget about the other person. It's easy to get caught up in the 'sex haze' and totally forget that there is another person sharing an intimate moment with you. Being able to exercise self-control is important here. Does this mean stopping your intimate interaction and asking your partner for permission with every single move you make? Maybe! Though it might sound ridiculous to some, it's important to check in throughout intimate encounters. *'Is this ok?' 'Do you like it when I do this?' 'Harder?' 'Softer' 'What would you like me to do?'* Asking these and other questions can be helpful in gauging a partner's level of comfort. Using critical thinking skills and adjusting your behavior based on your partner's comfort level is a major part of this equation. Making a conscious effort to listen and shift your focus to your partner, not just focusing on your own pleasure, will help you stay present and connected to your partner.

"As a Sex Educator and Sex Worker, consent is extremely important. For me my 'Aha moment' was giving my clients permission to consent to their kinks, allowing themselves to enjoy an activity they may have never allowed themselves to enjoy before. I feel joy in providing a safe environment for a person through my sex work, and providing education for the client to enjoy themselves safely."

- Miss Quin, Sex Educator/Adult Performer
Twitter @ThatMissQuin

Consent comic written and illustrated by Tikva Wolf, first
published in Greatist Magazine
KimchiCuddles.com

The first time I was raped, it was unintentional.
It was also the first time I was kissed. I was 14
or 15, and he was several years older. We were
kissing, but then he suddenly reached a hand up
my skirt. I'm sure he just thought he was "getting
lucky" because I didn't say anything, but I had
completely shut down and was trapped in a silent
panic as I watched the rest unfold. It was like one
of those dreams where you're just completely
paralyzed while the monster is closing in on you.

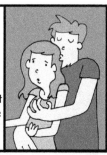

So, call me sometime?

How did this happen?

He had no idea I'd felt violated. He'd been taught
to "just go for it". When he was done, he asked
me if we could start dating. No one had taught
him about panic freeze responses, how to ask
his partners for consent, or how to notice when
they were actually enjoying themselves. This
example of unintentional rape is depressingly
common. We think of sexual assault as a thing
happening in dark alleys at the hands of villains,
but a lot of it happens in our own bedrooms at
the hands of people who didn't want to harm us.

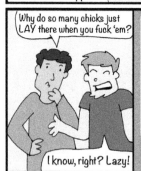

Why do so many chicks just
LAY there when you fuck 'em?

I know, right? Lazy!

Violations happen when people aren't
aware of how to truly listen for consent.
Consent never sounds (or looks) like
someone going limp and just laying
there staring off into nothing. If your
partner is just silently laying there and
seems spaced out, that might just be
how they are, but....

IT'S VERY LIKELY THAT
YOU'RE RAPING THEM.

When confronted with a threat, we often go into FIGHT or FLIGHT survival strategies, but when our brain assesses that we are likely unable to defeat the threat in battle or outrun it, we often go into FREEZE instead.

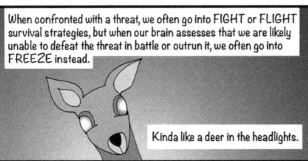

Kinda like a deer in the headlights.

This is called dissociation, and feels like being disconnected from what's actually happening. It is extremely common (especially for young women, but anyone of any age or gender is susceptible) to dissociate during sex when someone feels powerless to prevent it from happening.

My body can't get away, but the rest of me CAN!

Realizing you might have done this to someone doesn't mean that you need to take on a huge pile of guilt and tattoo RAPIST on your forehead to avoid all human contact. Instead, realizing that you violated someone can be an opportunity to learn how to be more aware in the future. By practicing being fully engaged when listening to your partner's verbal and nonverbal cues, you can become more thoroughly aware of their level of enthusiasm, and be an active part of healing our culture!

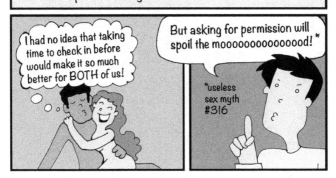

I had no idea that taking time to check in before would make it so much better for BOTH of us!

But asking for permission will spoil the mooooooooooooooood! *

*useless sex myth #316

Checking in only takes seconds, builds trust, ensures everyone's having a good time, and can prevent loved ones from enduring trauma. When everyone is actually making a conscious decision to participate, that's when things really get sexy! Not to mention, there are some VERY sexy ways to ask for consent!

Nervously avoiding asking each other what you truly want to share is what ACTUALLY spoils the mood. Talking about all your hidden desires is what enables you to share the types of experiences you want to.

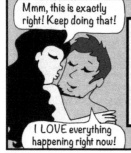

I'm so happy you told me your fantasies! I had no idea and I'm so excited to try it with you!

I'm so happy I said something!

Mmm, this is exactly right! Keep doing that!

Listening for consent isn't just waiting for a "yes," and then charging forward. It's cultivating an ongoing awareness of the degree of mutual enthusiasm for what's being shared. BOTH partners are responsible for cultivating this type of ongoing awareness.

I LOVE everything happening right now!

Listening for consent means being curious about your partners' experience every step of the way, both verbally as well as non-vernbally, and noticing if they get quiet, still, or stiff.

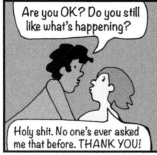

Are you OK? Do you still like what's happening?

Holy shit. No one's ever asked me that before. THANK YOU!

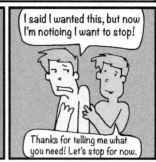

I said I wanted this, but now I'm noticing I want to stop!

Thanks for telling me what you need! Let's stop for now.

Consent is clear, communicated, enthusiastic, ongoing, and can be revoked at any time. If something stops feeling good for one of you, stop doing it! If your partner feels uneasy, take a break!

Talk about boundaries and preferences about touch BEFORE initiating a new kind of touch. Getting consent to kiss ISN'T getting consent to grope anywhere else, and vice versa! Don't worry about sounding corny. If they're into it, anything you ask will probably sound super sexy.

I'm really enjoying kissing your beautiful lips. May I also kiss your amazing breasts?

Mmm Hmm!!

Consent is a mutual, enthusiastic, ongoing HELL YES about everything that is happening. Be aware of the feelings in yourself and and also in the person(s) you're engaging with. Listening includes looking for nonverbal cues. A person can communicate non-consent by looking uncomfortable, going limp, getting quiet, squirming, or crying.

Ask questions along the way and give full attention to the answer!

Do you like this?

Do you want to take a break?

How do you want to be touched right now?

Hold on. I want to check in to see if this still feels good

I'm so happy that it matters to you how I feel!

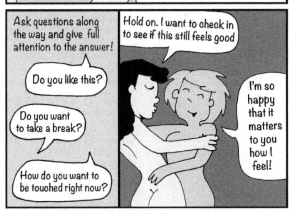

Remember to check in with YOURSELF as well. If you feel any nervousness about your "performance," SLOW DOWN so you're able to be aware of what's going on with your partner. It's completely OK to take a break to come back to yourself!

Consent involves checking in before, during, AND after. Talking about your shared experience afterward is an important step in learning what your partner would like to share with you, and gives them the chance to talk about anything stressful that might have came up by surprise.

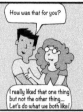

Certain factors affect a person's ability to give consent. Anyone who is underage, unconscious, or making decisions under the influence of substances is unable to give consent,

PERIOD.

Power imbalances also can also impact the ability of someone to feel comfortable to say no, ask for what they want, or engage in fully consensual activities. It is important to be aware of what privileges you have and take extra care when listening for verbal as well as nonverbal cues of distress.

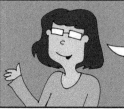

FUN FACT: Unless you grew up in a forest raised by wood elves and haven't ever come in contact with other humans before, you HAVE been influenced by our culture, and therefore have been affected by cultural privileges. Paying attention to how this affects the people around you is an important aspect of truly cultivating consent culture!

Practicing being aware of your partners' experience is one of the strongest ways you can nourish consent culture while building a foundation of trust between you and your partner. When you practice noticing your partners' verbal and nonverbal cues and listening with ALL your senses, you can open up a delicious explosion of succulent sensuality you never knew was possible!

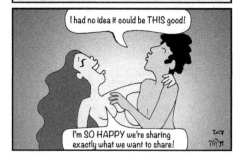

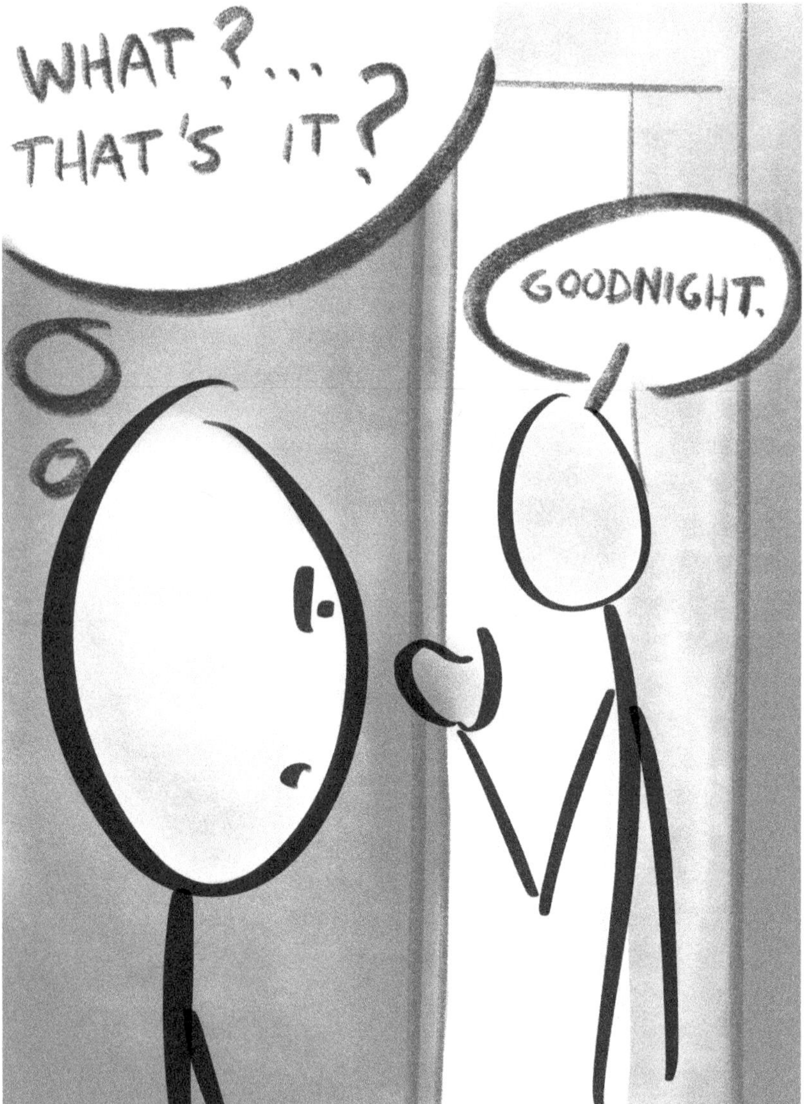
WHAT?... THAT'S IT?
GOODNIGHT.

The Assumption of Intercourse

Never assume anything as far as sex and intimate encounters are concerned. By default there is often an assumption that sex is the only option when it comes to dating and intimacy. There is an assumption that if someone wants to kiss, that automatically means that they want to have sex. Maybe your intimate partner is currently choosing to abstain from intercourse. Consider that they might be interested in having sex with you, but they only want to kiss right now. The right choice is the choice where both participants feel comfortable. If you are not okay with someone's boundaries, they may not be a good fit for you. If you see potential with someone, be patient and respect their boundaries. Knowing your boundaries and having a YES/NO/MAYBE conversation can be helpful in not making assumptions around intimate choices.

"The current movement started by Tarana Burke, with the long overdue social dialogue on consent, is just the beginning of a larger consciousness. We are a society that desperately needs to look at the subtleties and intersections of power. This extends to questions of gender, representation, political realities, and social conscience. My hope is that as we extend this dialogue, we will find more accurate words to describe the constellations of experiences, which shine beyond the narratives we so often explain the world by."

- tenerDuende

"Consent is a continuous conversation. It goes beyond trusting and knowing another person. It involves understanding what the potential actions and consequences are. It involves knowing enough about one's body and mind to claim ownership of them and to explore with them. It involves centering pleasure as a fundamental aspect of life. Speaking as a Survivor of childhood sexual assault, I have these continuous conversations with myself often. With new friends, new partners, and new situations, it has been useful for me to think of consent in this way...as an ongoing conversation with levels of negotiation. To have full agency over my body, mind, and pleasure, means that no one can touch me or make me feel less than my glorious sea goddess self."

- Goddess Cecilia, Sexuality & Pleasure Educator
GoddessCecilia.com

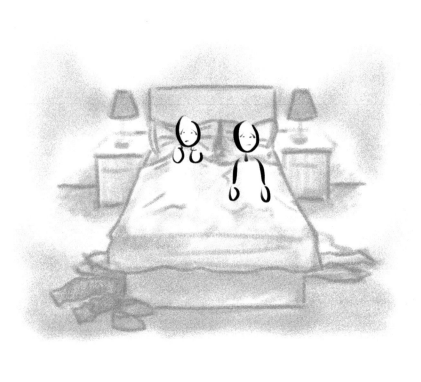

Using Positive Reinforcement After An Encounter

In intimate scenarios, there can be situations where someone you like, and possibly respect, might misread and/or not be tuned in to your non-verbal cues and unintentionally crosses your boundaries. This is in no way meant to give boundary-crossers a 'pass,' but if someone does cross your boundaries, and you would like to give them another chance, ongoing communication is crucial. In some cases, it is very possible that the person who crossed your boundaries might not even be aware that any harm was done, or that you might have felt (or still feel) uneasy about a past encounter with them. If you are able and want to give them another chance, it's imperative that you discuss what improvements can be made going forward.

These conversations can feel uncomfortable if you've never had a conversation about boundaries with someone, especially if that someone is an intimate partner. Here are a few phrases that can be helpful when having a conversation about boundaries with someone you would like to keep interacting with. These phrases are meant to encourage positive and constructive improvements, while keeping the shaming to a minimum.

"It would be great if you would..."
"It makes me super excited when you..."
"I'd really love it if you'd…"
"I really love it when you…"
"It makes me feel really comfortable when you…"
"Instead of _____, could you/we try _____?"
"Is there anything you'd like me to do differently next time?"

Positive reinforcement can be very helpful! Tell your partner what you love that they did after they did it!!

In this new age of consent, it's important that you have a general idea of what your own boundaries are before entering into consensual interactions and relationships. Your YES/NO/MAYBE list will help you set boundaries with everyone in your life. It will act as a tangible starting point to help you consciously choose positive people, situations, and interactions. By being clear about what your boundaries are in different scenarios, it will be much easier to know when one of your boundaries has been crossed. Keep in mind that your boundaries might change, morph, evolve, or progress as you get to know different people and are in different situations. Just always take a moment to check in with yourself so that you know what feels right to you during each encounter and with each individual. Also keep in mind that even if you have a specific boundary with a partner, you are always at liberty to adjust that previous boundary based upon anything from a mood shift, level of comfort, a change in your partner's behavior, because it's Monday... whatever!

It's your choice to change your boundaries and, because they are *your* boundaries, you have the power to change them at your discretion. If your boundaries do change, it can be helpful information to let those you are interacting with know that your boundaries have changed, so that you are on the same page. This will help lessen confusion and the potential for misunderstandings or negative interactions with others. If you are not ok with a partner's boundaries, they might not be a good choice of partner for you. Find someone whose boundaries and emotional intelligence are more in alignment with yours rather than trying to change, shame, or guilt them into adjusting their level of comfort. Conversely, if you feel that someone is not respecting your boundaries or has a different level of emotional intelligence, consider moving on to find someone who fully accepts you and your YES/NO/MAYBEs.

"I never had any formalized sexual health education when I was in school, let alone anything on consent. I didn't even know consent during sexual encounters was a thing until I stumbled into the women's center by accident in college. Though I was never formally taught about consent, growing up I noticed that many women and girls had sex that they did not want to have and that sexual pleasure was never an option. I wanted to change that in my own life, so I talked about sex before having sex, learned about what made me sexually happy, and took my time discussing boundaries with my partner."

- Sadia Arshad, Educator with HEART Women and Girls
HeartWomenAndGirls.org

Consenting Once Doesn't Mean Lifetime Access

It is imperative that you aim to get consent during each encounter with each person that you will be intimate with. Circumstances, feelings, and boundaries may have changed from the first encounter to the next. Assumptions should not be made about a partner's consent between encounters. Avoiding assumptions when it comes to kissing, touching, and any other intimate contact helps to protect you from any misunderstandings or boundary missteps. You do not know what has happened in someone's life since the last time you saw them. It's also important to remember that some people might not be looking for exactly the same interaction that you may have had in the past – for various reasons. Just as people's moods change...just as you most likely don't want to eat the same thing for every meal every day, people's feelings and desires change. Don't make assumptions.

Beyond that, it's important to be aware that you might not know what else that person has going on in their life at that moment. Maybe they are dealing with something serious and an intimate encounter might make them feel smothered. Maybe they are simply in a different place in their life than they were during your previous encounter and that has caused them to make different choices. It's important not to make someone feel 'wrong' about respecting their own feelings and boundaries. No one should ever feel forced into an intimate encounter. If someone from your past doesn't want to have a specific interaction with you, give them space and don't take it personally.

It's also important to note that just because someone might not want to, for example, kiss you like they did before, it doesn't mean that they want nothing to do with you... but then again maybe it does. This is why communication is so important. There might be some instances where someone would rather cuddle with you rather than engage in a heavy make-out session. There might be times when your former cuddle buddy might not want to be kissed or cuddled and simply wants to be left alone. Maybe they don't want to be touched but they'd like to talk. There are so many possibilities here. Communicate. Don't Make Assumptions. Don't Take Anything Personally.

Each encounter should be treated with respect, and consent should be given in each circumstance. Consent is not fixed... it is fluid. Depending on the agreements of each participant, the consent parameters could vary, but there should be a clear sign that each party is on board with regards to specific acts and during each encounter. However, we all have different moods and are in different places in our lives at any given moment. Sometimes we might need more care and consideration. Sometimes we might not be 'in the mood' for a kiss or a touch. It's important to acknowledge that because our individual experiences are varied and our feelings, desires, and comfort levels can change, it's important to check in with your potential partners regularly throughout a specific interaction and from encounter to encounter.

A Word About Stealthing

Respect your partner's request to use protection. Removing a condom or any other means of protection during intimate encounters violates the consensual agreement the two of you made. If you are not in agreement about altering the agreed upon means of protection, that is a non-consensual decision.

CHAPTER 8

Survivor Support

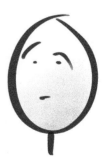

Every 98 seconds another American is sexually assaulted.

rainn.org

"Building a consent culture is inherently related to developing a sex-positive culture. People socialized as female are conditioned to believe that in order to be 'good,' they have to remain 'virginal.' If they show sexual interest, they're labeled 'sluts.' People socialized as men are taught that in order to be 'good,' they have to get sex. They're also taught that persistence is valuable and not to take NO for an answer. It's no wonder we see this trend of masculine folks pursuing femmes, femmes resisting, and masculine people trying to push the envelope. Want to promote a consent culture? Start by making it okay for femmes to want and have sex so that masculine types can trust that when his potential partner says NO, she really means it, and he, in turn, doesn't push her boundaries to prove his masculinity by pressuring her."

- Atrina, Relationship Educator
Atrina, NYC

Why Survivors Don't Speak Up

I've had so many conversations with people who have questioned this 'new shift' in awareness around consent. Some have even gone as far as to ask *why now* and *why didn't people speak up sooner.* Just because people are speaking up now doesn't mean that it hasn't been a problem for many years. Oftentimes when someone does speak out about their boundaries being crossed, more questions are posed to the boundary-crossee than to the boundary-crosser. Blaming or shaming an individual for being violated for any reason is like blaming the victim of a dog bite for getting bitten, or blaming someone who had their valuables stolen for allowing the theft to happen. Empathy is important here. No one deserves to have their boundaries violated. Period.

There are numerous reasons why people choose to stay silent about harassment, abuse, and assault. These reasons include, but are not limited to…

1) Fear Of Not Being Believed

Sometimes people aren't believed when they speak out about a violation that has happened to them. It is common for the survivor to be blamed for their behavior rather than people being concerned about their well-being. The fear of this happening is one reason why people choose to suffer in silence after a violation occurs.

2) Loss Of Privacy

The accuser might not want to put themselves in the public eye to be talked about, and possibly publicly harassed, ridiculed, or threatened for coming forward - especially if the person being accused is well-known, well-respected, or famous. If the public knows the accused, the lesser-known accuser can become collateral damage in the process of coming forward with their story.

3) Reliving The Incident

Every time a specific incident is repeated out loud, the victim can have the horrific experience of reliving the trauma all over again. Why would anyone want to voluntarily go through that experience again? It is an extremely difficult decision for someone to speak out, sometimes repeatedly, about traumatic events. For some survivors, trying to move on and try to forget the incident is the 'best' option, but, for others, this is not easy and might be next to impossible.

4) Fear Of Intimidation Or Violence

In certain cases, the accused might even intimidate or threaten the accuser if they speak up about what has happened. Even if it's an empty threat, it is a very scary notion to someone who might feel vulnerable and has already gone through a traumatic experience. Realistically, the accuser may not know what the accused is capable of and what lengths they will go to keep the them silent.

5) Fear Of Intimidation Or Violence Against Others

Imagine that an accuser already feels threatened and isn't sure what the boundary-crosser is capable of. What if the accused then threatens the accuser's family or friends? That adds another layer of intimidation and fear to the situation. Some accusers choose to stay silent to protect others that they care about – in case the accused is capable of following through with the threats they have made.

6) Fear Of Losing Job Or Income

Ironically, because people have adverse reactions directed at accusers who speak out about personal consent-related incidents, coming forward can sometimes have a negative effect on their job – just because they chose not to stay silent. A lot of the high-profile cases in the news have involved high-earning individuals. The stakes become higher if someone isn't living a life of financial privilege. The fear of losing one's income increases if the incident actually occurred in the workplace. If someone isn't wealthy and has had their boundaries crossed, the decision to 'just quit' becomes exponentially more difficult. This job might be their only source of income.

7) Fear Of Losing Friends/Community

If an incident has occurred within a tight-knit group of people, it can feel scary to come forward and speak about someone in that community who has breached another's boundaries. It can be incredibly intimidating to tell other members of a community that an admired person in the community has violated someone's boundaries.

8) Fear That Justice Will Not Be Served

It is not a given that justice will be served, if you file a police report and take someone to court. Not everyone has faith in the justice system, and the system does not guarantee justice. Plus, the legal process can be lengthy and costly. For some, it feels easier to avoid the process of getting the law involved and all that entails.

9) Lack Of Funds To Hire Quality Legal Representation

It takes money and resources to get a lawyer, to pay for a lawyer, and to go through the legal process. Not everyone has the money to 'just get a lawyer and sue.' Not everyone has access to quality legal representation. This can be a massive barrier that prevents people from pursuing legal justice.

10) Intimidation By Powerful Individuals

If someone is well known or famous, even more complicated factors can enter into the picture. Several of the aforementioned fears can come into play and there might be enablers who work with these powerful individuals to help keep these incidents 'secret,' allowing patterns to continue. There might be attempts to 'pay off' individuals for their silence. In extreme cases, intimidation tactics and threats of destroying careers are legitimate possibilities.

In all of these cases, there is the very real experience of the victim having 'double the trauma' after coming forward. Not only did they experience something ranging from unpleasant to traumatic, but the aftermath of dealing with public's perception and possible harassment makes the decision to come forward much more difficult. These are just a few reasons why people choose not to come forward when their boundaries have been violated.

"Hopefully, America is living through a fundamental culture shift - a shift away from sex as conquest, seduction as salesmanship, and male entitlement as a 'grin-and-bear-it' reality... a shift toward sex as an honest, collaborative celebration; toward seduction as a playfully mutual ritual dance. If we're really lucky, we'll see the next generation develop mating rituals based on an assumption of agency and autonomy on both sides, based on an embracing of our sexual selves as something cherished and joyful rather than something dangerous and shameful. I believe we're witnessing the grotesque dying throes of conquest culture. I believe we're witnessing the rise of the sexually empowered woman."

- Cassie Brighter, Author/Speaker
CassieBrighter.com

"Consent always seems such an elusive concept to so many. The idea that you can take and hold power over someone else's body, against their will, shouldn't even be up for debate. The problem has always been about power and its distribution. Sexual assault, after all, is not about sex, it's about power, and those who exert their will over others to prove something to themselves."

- Dr. Donna Oriowo, Speaker/Sex Educator/Therapist
www.AnnodRight.com

After An Incident

There is no 'one way' to feel, act, or proceed after a boundary-crossing incident. It can take time to process the specific details. Some survivors might not know where to go or what next steps to take. Though everyone's healing process will be unique, there are some important things that can be helpful for a survivor. Here are some possible initial options...

1. Get To A Safe Place & Tell Someone That You Trust

Your safety is the most important thing! If your boundaries were crossed at a party, event, bar, school, or in the workplace, do what you can to get away from that location and get to a place where you feel safe. That safe place could be your own home, a friend's home, or a shelter. Once you've gotten to a safe space, share what happened with someone you trust. This could be a community member, friend, dorm/resident assistant, teacher, counselor, family member, or anyone else that you feel you can confide in. Telling your story to a trusted individual can be helpful emotionally, and also if you decide to report the incident to authorities later on.

2. Restorative Justice

Once again, if you are a part of an intentional community and your boundaries were crossed by another member, restorative justice is a possible option. Restorative justice can be a solution for those who want to continue to be a part of a community and are able to participate in the process of understanding and healing with the help of this close-knit social circle. This is only possible if all participants are willing to be active participants in the process.

3. Reporting An Incident To Authorities

There might be some cases where it is appropriate to report an incident to authorities. It's up to the individual to decide if this is the best course of action for them. Starting the legal process can be time-consuming, expensive, and emotionally exhausting, but it can also be cathartic and an opportunity to receive some level of justice. Everyone has to choose a resolution that feels best for them and, in some cases, that solution might be to file a police report against a boundary-crosser.

4. Counseling/Therapy

Seeking professional help can be an effective way to start the healing process. A professional therapist or counselor can be of assistance in the journey of healing physical and emotional trauma. Anger, fear, sadness, and so many other emotions can be part of the healing process. It's important to remember that anger directed at your boundary-pusher ultimately takes energy away from your life. Learning new tools from an objective professional can be a helpful option to move forward after a traumatic incident.

5. Ongoing Self-Care

What is going to help you in your journey to heal? What steps can you take to put your care first? Moving forward, it's important to check in with yourself regularly to be aware of your level of comfort with others. This can include getting comfortable enforcing your boundaries and taking time for yourself whenever you feel you need to. This might mean going home early when out with friends because something or someone made you feel uncomfortable. It could also mean taking a total break from social interactions for a while – including dating. Maybe there is a local survivors' group that could be helpful. Take as much time as you need to go through the healing process.

The Impact Of Violating Someone's Consent

We typically assess things in terms of, 'How can I get what I want?' It's important to able to take ourselves out of the 'ME' place for a moment and think about how our actions impact those around us. It has been normalized to aggressively go after what we want sexually and do whatever it takes to get it. As a society, we are very egocentric, and this mindset can lead to boundary-crossing and individuals not taking others into consideration.

Whether your boundary crossing was intentional or unintentional, it has made an impact on the other person involved. Your actions have a ripple effect. Your actions ARE a big deal. There might not be physical scars, but the emotional scars and related associations to certain actions, behaviors, sensations, and/or touches can be very deep. Some people require years of counseling and therapy to undo that harm and learn how to trust people and walk comfortably in the world again. Certain types of trauma can change someone forever. Just because you don't think your actions weren't a big deal, doesn't mean that it's true. Here are some statistics from Anti-Sexual Violence Organization **rainn. org** that show the impact of sexual assault. *Visit **rainn.org** for more detailed statistics.*

- *94% of women who are raped experience symptoms of post-traumatic stress disorder (PTSD) during the two weeks following the rape.*

- *30% of women report symptoms of PTSD 9 months after the rape.*

- *33% of women who are raped contemplate suicide.*

- *Approximately 70% of rape or sexual assault victims experience moderate to severe distress, a larger percentage than for any other violent crime.*

Your actions can change someone's life forever and possibly affect all their future interactions. Your actions not only affect the person you are interacting with, but their friends and family by association. That is the impact we are talking about. It's going to a crowded bar and no longer seeing it as a fun experience; it becomes a room full of strangers who don't have your best interests at heart, who might do you harm. It's going to the office every day and having your job become secondary to managing emotions or avoiding interactions with a boss or coworker. It's going on a date and not seeing it as a fun and exciting opportunity to get to know a potential partner; instead, it becomes a stressful encounter with a stranger who wants to take advantage of you because they only see you and your body for pleasure purposes.

We all have a responsibility to be conscious of our actions, exercise self-control, and not abuse our power and privilege when interacting with others. How you exist in this world will affect not only your life and legacy, but the life and legacy of those you interact with. What do you want your legacy to be? How do you want to be seen? How do you want to be perceived? Is getting what you want more important than someone else's boundaries potentially being violated? Is boundary-pushing worth litigation? Are you willing to possibly give up your freedom to get what you want by pushing someone's boundaries? It is THAT serious.

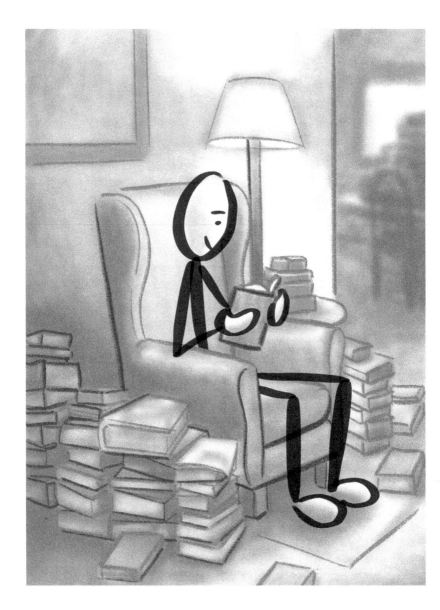

Resources

There is no shame in asking for help. The following list provides various resources for sexual assault survivors, sexual harassment support, suicide prevention, and substance abuse support, as well as sexual education and healthy relationship resources. This list should not take the place of medical advice. If you have specific concerns or a situation in which you require professional or medical advice, you should consult an appropriately trained and qualified specialist.

AL-ANON
Support for Families and Friends of Alcoholics
AL-ANON.org

Alcoholics Anonymous
International Fellowship of Individuals Who Seek Help with an Alcohol Addiction
AA.org

The Betty Ford Center
The Nation's Largest Non-Profit Treatment Provider for Individuals, Communities, and Families Affected by Addiction to Alcohol and Other Drugs
800-434-7518
HazeldenBettyFord.org

Break The Cycle
Inspiring Young People 12-24 to Build Healthy Relationships And Create A Culture Without Abuse
BreakTheCycle.org

Center Against Sexual Assault
Promoting Safe and Healthy Relationships Based on Dignity, Respect, Compassion, and Equality
866-373-8300
SWCASA.org

CoDA - Co-Dependents Anonymous International
A Fellowship of Men and Women Whose Common Purpose is to Develop Healthy Relationships and Break the Cycle of Co-Dependence
CoDA.org

Date Safe Project
Providing Workshops and Resources for Consent, Bystander Intervention, and Survivor Support
DateSafeProject.org

End Rape On Campus
Works to End Campus Sexual Violence Through Direct Support of Survivors and Their Communities; Prevention Through Education; and Policy Reform at the Campus, Local, State, and Federal Levels
EndRapeOnCampus.com

Geeks For Consent
Dedicated to Creating a More Inclusive and Safe Convention Culture
GeeksForConsent.org

Know The Signs
Suicide Prevention Site Designed to Help Start a Conversation with and Provide Resources for Someone Who Has Suicidal Thoughts
1-800-273-8255
SuicideIsPreventable.org

Men Can Stop Rape
Mobilizing Men to Use Their Strength for Creating Cultures Free from Violence, Especially Men's Violence Against Women
MenCanStopRape.org

National Domestic Violence Hotline
Providing One-on-One Support Including Crisis Intervention, Options for Next Steps, and Direct Connection to Resources for Immediate Safety
1-800-799-SAFE (7233)
TheHotline.org

National Sexual Violence Resource Center
Providing Leadership in Preventing And Responding to Sexual Violence Through Collaboration, Sharing and Creating Resources, and Promoting Research
NSVRC.org

NO MORE
Dedicated to Ending Domestic Violence and Sexual Assault by Increasing Awareness, Inspiring Action, and Fueling Culture Change
NoMore.org

RAINN/National Sexual Abuse Hotline
"Largest Anti-Sexual Violence Organization in North America"
800-656-HOPE (4673)
RAINN.org

Scarleteen
Online Sex Ed, Sexuality, and Relationships Resource for Teens & Emerging Adults
Scarleteen.com

Sex And Stats
A Statistics-Based Blog Focused on Sex and Sexuality
SexAndStats.com

SWOP - Sex Worker Outreach Program
Social justice network dedicated to the fundamental human rights of people involved in the sex trade and their communities, focusing on ending violence and stigma through education and advocacy.
New.SWOPUSA.org

SIECUS-Sexuality Information and Education Council of the United States
Sexuality and Information Council of the United States
SIECUS.org

Time's Up Legal Defense Fund
Legal Assistance for Individuals Who Have Sexual Harassment or Related Retaliation in the Workplace
TimesUpNow.com

The Trevor Project
Suicide Prevention Resource for LGBTQ Youth
TheTrevorProject.org

EPILOGUE

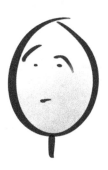

The culture around consent, intimacy, and boundaries is in a major state of revolution and evolution. Because survivors are coming forward and sharing their stories on a massive scale, there is more awareness of this societal problem. The next step is to create and implement education and solutions. Survivor support needs to be a priority, but how do we rehabilitate boundary-crossers? For some, consent-based education can be enough to change behavior. For others, more severe consequences might be necessary to change their behavior. What should the corresponding consequences be for each scenario? Serious situations may need to be handled in a court of law.

New consent-based strategies can be learned. I am hopeful that we can unlearn the idea that getting what you want comes at the expense of someone else's safety or comfort, and embrace the concept of creating mutually respectful interactions in which care is taken and everyone involved benefits. Now is the beginning of a major shift in the way we interact with each other –hopefully that change will be significantly more respectful and consensual.

The topic of consent should be treated as an ongoing conversation. I believe that we can find solutions and create major change...together.

NOTES

THANK YOU

**Thank you to everyone who contributed to make this
book possible!**